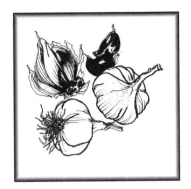

Your Guide To Standardized Herbal Products

By REBECCA FLYNN, M.S. and
MARK ROEST
Forward by DANIEL MOWREY, Ph.D.

ONE WORLD PRESS

January 1995, First Edition

© One World Press, 1995

ISBN: 0-9644958-0-5
Library of Congress: 94-80040

Printed in The U.S.

Layout, Typography and Cover Design: Shukyo Lin Rainey

One World Press
601 Granada Drive
Prescott, AZ 86301

TABLE
OF CONTENTS

PREFACE

Herbs have been used throughout time for cooking and as a primary tool for maintaining health and for aiding in the recovery of disease. The ancient Egyptians, Greeks, Chinese, and Native American Indians have revered and respected the powers of Nature and her herbal kingdom. Socrates said "Let food be thy medicine."

With the scientific medical revolution of the twentieth century, many of the age-old remedies from folk medicine were discarded in the wake of powerful, modern drugs. These drugs however have not fulfilled their promise of magical cures. Their use has been limited by severe life-threatening side effects. Many of these drugs do not heal people of their ills, instead they only temporarily (but quickly) remove all symptoms of disease. But this symptomatic relief in no way means an alleviation of disease. To the contrary, the disease is pushed further in and quietly but inexorably moves forward destroying more and more of a person's health.

Furthermore, it is in this symptomatic relief that the greatest danger of all exists, that of the loss of patient self-responsibility. With the instantaneous relief offered by the modern pharma-copoeias, no longer do people need to worry about what they eat or drink, or how much they abuse their bodies or how much exercise if any they need to do. Nor is there any motivation to clean up dangerous lifestyles and change unhealthy habits. There's always a little white or red or yellow pill that will magically make all problems go away.

Slowly, however, people are beginning to understand the problems with our "quick-fix" attitude toward health and disease. They realize that they are not getting better despite the pills and their temporary relief of headaches, stomach aches, gas, and constipation. They still feel tired all the time. They huff and puff after walking up a flight of stairs. They get depressed before their periods. They still have cramps every month. They still get chest pains. They're not standing as tall as in the past. And its not only small problems either. They have an attack of kidney stones. They get cirrhosis and liver failure. They have a heart attack or a stroke out of the blue. They get cancer.

The lack of help from modern medicine has led to the resurgence during the past decade in the popularity of herbal medicine along with nutrition and holistic medicine. Modern science and technology have now been put to use studying the herbal pharmacopoeia. Enormous quantities of information has been generated validating the ancient folk remedies. Ancient techniques of extracting herbs have found value as well. The ancient Greeks and Egyptians made decoctions, infusions, tinctures, and syrups from their herbs in order to make them easier to swallow at the correct dose and in many cases made them more effective than the raw leaf or bark. Even pleasant tasting teas, such as chamomile or licorice root were found to have physiological effects, calming people or reducing spasms, alleviating anxiety, treating ulcers, reducing inflammation, or helping reduce joint pains.

Numerous scientific experiments have led to the identification and purification of many of the unique compounds of various herbs. Science has found ways of purifying and concentrating the herbs and their unique compounds. From this technology has come the ability to standardize herbal preparations to a particular quantity of unique compounds and to insure that the correct species of plants at the correct level of potency are used in the processing.

Standardization has the ability to assure the correct species identification of herb plant material and the relative strength of the finished herbal product. Standardization does not furnish definition of phytopharmaceutical activity as defined from a traditional herbal perspective.

Standardization insures that you know what is in the product, know its potency, and know the correct amount to consume. Standardization guarantees that the product is made from good quality, unsubstituted, and correct species of plants with no contaminants. Quality extraction companies take additional precautions with their herbs to ensure the highest quality final product. The quality of their raw materials is judged based on many other analyses such as taste, smell, microbiological analysis, pH, solubility and appearance in addition to standardization.

In some case the primary active ingredient is unknown or there may be several active ingredients. By standardizing the herb based on one "marker" ingredient with care taken not to alter the proportions of all the ingredients in relation to the marker, you can obtain virtually identical batches of products. This consistency is extremely important for physicians and professional caregivers who can treat patients and achieve consistent results. Standardization and Guaranteed Potency have made it possible to validate the efficacy of herbal preparations which is the beginning step towards scientific acceptance.

ABOUT THE BOOK

This book gives detailed descriptions of the major standardized and Guaranteed Potency medical herbs currently available to the informed practitioner. The book has been developed to provide the professional in the field with up-to-date information regarding standardized herbs which are available in the market.

The book includes a quick reference guide detailing common conditions and herbs that have been found to be helpful. The chapter for

i

each herb includes a description of the herb and the type of plant, its natural habitat, and traditional medicinal uses. The active ingredients of each plant are discussed and their pharmacological actions in the body. The currently published medical and research studies are summarized under active properties. Each chapter includes common directions for use of the standardized extracts and known cautions or contraindications associated with the herb. Finally, the normal processing procedures used to extract the herb and standardize it to its active ingredients are briefly mentioned. The information about each herb has been obtained from a wide range of sources, including scientific medical papers, published research studies, medical text books, and modern herbals. Most of the references are included with each herb. More extended reference lists can be obtained from bibliographies of the listed references.

We are privileged to have Dr. Daniel Mowrey write the introduction to our book. Dr. Mowrey has published extensively in well known journals, ranging from "The Herbalist" to the prestigious medical journal the British "Lancet." Dr. Mowrey's background includes a Ph.D. in psychology and psychopharmacology from Brigham Young University, with related studies in biochemistry and biology. He has served on the faculty of Brigham Young University and was the Director of Research at Amtec Industries and Director of the Mountainwest Institute of Herbal Science. He is currently on the staff of the American Phytotherapy Research Laboratory (APRL). Dr. Mowrey has been directly involved with toxicology tests and efficacy studies on numerous herbs and herbal formulations.

The book is only a guide to research that has been done to date. More research needs to be performed to increase our knowledge of herbs and of the great potential of herbal medicine.

SELECTION OF STANDARDIZED HERBS

The development of standardized herbs is relatively new. Initiated by a 1992 change in European Law, Guaranteed Potency or measured dosage is quickly changing the face of herbal medicine. Doctors can now prescribe herbal treatments with confidence of consistent results. Standards are not always defined in the same way. The selection of a standard constituent to measure in an herb varies among competitive companies. The herb Valerian has been measured by three different standards—valerenic acid, volative oils, or valeopotriates. The development of a standard is expensive and often there are scientific disagreements as to the best standard. In this book, we have tried to identify the most useful standards.

Standardizing usually involves extraction, which adds three benefits: (1) the constituents of extracted herbs are more easily absorbed than when they are locked up in cellulose walls; the herbs are essentially partially pre-digested; (2) more stringent quality control procedures are brought to bear on the herb; (3) the total volume of the herb is reduced, making it more convenient to package, ship and use.

The professional should look for the best combination of three variables in selecting a product: (1) the strength of the key constituents; (2) the balance of the other constituents; and (3) the price per dose.

The weighting assigned to each variable depends on the nature of the herb. Most herbs have very complex actions, with many complementing and balancing constituents. It is important to assure that all of the constiuents are present in their normal ratios when these have been shown to depend on one or a few key constituents, while the rest of the herb is much less important. In some cases, constituents are deliberately eliminated, to prevent toxicity, irritation, or dilution of the desired effect.

The price of herbal extracts reflect the cost of the bulk herb, the ratio of bulk herb to final extract, the cost of processing the herb into an extract, and the relative value of the extract in the market, based on its therapeutic contribution. For example, Ginkgo Biloba 24% is a 50:1 concentration "purified" extract, in which some constituents are highly controlled. Clinical use indicated that a total extract at 8:1 concentration (about 1/6 of 50:1) did not produce all the results that the 24% extract does, even at much more than 6 times the quantity, so the 8:1's low price is *not* a bargain.

As an example in the other direction, Dong Quai works very well as a simple soup, and the quality of the herb strongly influences the quality of the extract. The most active constituents have not been conclusively identified, and wellmade "total" extracts with low concentrations are likely to carry a greater percentage of the original constituents than highly concentrated extracts. In this case, the lower price truly is a bargain.

The final issue that determines the price of extracts is a combination of skill, efficiency, and economies of scale or labor the manufacturer provides. Breakthroughs occur frequently, as members of the industry share their findings with their customers or suppliers, who use the information to seek an even better approach in their own work.

INTRODUCTION

by Daniel Mowrey, Ph.D.

During the past decade or so we have witnessed a phenomenal rise in the popularity of herbal medicines in America. We have been in the process of rediscovering our medical roots and are finding that folk medicine has now found scientific validation. An enormous quantity of scientific information has originated from overseas and slowly has been transferred to America. Indeed since the publication of *The Scientific Validation of Herbal Medicine*, I have noticed an increasingly greater degree of public sophistication concerning herbal medicine in the United States.

Recent developments in the European market can only be described as revolutionary. We have been forced to discard the almost universally accepted theoretical limitation that any given herbal preparation was limited in effectiveness and potency by several factors: growing conditions, including soil, fertilization and insect control; climatic conditions, such as rainfall and temperature; harvesting procedures, including when and how; curing procedures; processing and preparation methods; packaging; storage; and shelf life.

European researchers discovered that most if not all of the variables listed above could be artificially controlled if you could standardize the amount of active principle in the final product. Then it would not matter if it took one bushel or 100 bushels of raw material — the end product would be the same. There were two hitches: knowing the active constituents of the plant, and then, being able to measure their presence in both the raw and final product. Actually, there was the third problem of establishing the standard in the first place, but that could be worked out while the basic research on the first two took place.

Efforts to solve the two main problems have been going on for several decades. Such research had paid off in several instances. Investigations continue in Germany, Italy, Russia, Switzerland, and France to find plants whose active constituents can be identified, standardized, and used to prepare the next generation of herbal products: *Guaranteed Potency Herbs*.

Guaranteed Potency Herbs are beginning to answer the often-heard complaint about herbal medicine: that one is never certain just how much active material is in any given batch. *Guaranteed Potency Herbs* are guaranteed by the manufacturer to contain at least the advertised amount of active ingredient and to contain the most potent and effective standardized forms of these active constituents. Science has validated during the past 20-30 years the safety and efficacy of several standardized herbal products. One can, therefore, have considerably more confidence in the reliability of such products.

One legitimate question is, does the use of *Guaranteed Potency Herbs* remove us one step from a wholistic approach to health? Being committed, myself, to wholistic health care, I have had to scrutinize the *Guaranteed Potency Herbs* approach very carefully. There are individuals who believe that any processing of herbal material is a violation of wholistic medicine. But those people should realize that brewing a tea, grinding, drying, and other "home-grown" procedures are all examples of processing. The encapsulated product is one more degree of processing, but so long as whole herb material is used, I think the capsule can safely be classified as wholistic. Extracts, whether alcohol, apple cider vinegar, glycerin, water, freeze-dried, or whatever, belong in the wholistic camp, as long as they are obtained directly from whole herb material and some attempt is made to retain the natural complement of active constituents.

Guaranteed Potency Herbs also begin and end with whole herb material. But in between, during the extraction process, the levels of certain key ingredients are measured and increased, if necessary. This procedure, if done unwisely, may result in the creation of an artificial imbalance between constituents. In order to prevent the alteration of any medicinal value that depends upon relative concentrations of active ingredients, much research is required to determine the nature of any key interactions among the active ingredients. Without that knowledge, the final product will simply be a best guess.

The determination of key interactions is generally obtained by testing various batches of herb material in physiological systems, recording which are most effective, and measuring the relative levels of all known constituents. Once this work has been done, researchers can attempt to alter subsequent batches of herb to match the relative levels of active constituents in the most effective batch. In other words the Guaranteed Potency Herbs concept recognizes the inherent variability in plant material, and hence the inherent variability in the effectiveness of plant material, and attempts to eliminate the variability from the end product.

The key to the *Guaranteed Potency Herb* concept is careful adherence to all research and processing stipulations required to insure that key ratios are not disturbed, but rather guaranteed, to be present. When those stipulations are followed, the resulting product conforms very well with the wholistic concept, and may be used by wholistic practitioners with greater confidence that raw material.

ABOUT THE AUTHORS...

REBECCA FLYNN

Rebecca Flynn is founder and president of Creative Nature Consulting which provides nutritional, scientific, and marketing expertise to a variety of natural vitamin and supplement companies in California, including Greater Continents, Ecological Formulas, and Optimal Nutrients. She received her MS in Immunology from the University of Pennsylvania and her BA from Bryn Mawr College, double majoring in Chemistry and Molecular/Cellular Biology. Ms. Flynn has studied nutrition extensively over the past 10 years. She has published several scientific articles and book chapters and attended numerous biomedical and nutritional seminars and conferences. Previous positions have included Director of Marketing and Sales at Cardiovascular Research, Ltd. and biomedical research assistant at Genentech, Inc.

MARK ROEST

Mark Roest has done product development work with dietary supplements for seven years, focusing on herbs and advanced nutrients. He helped bring the *Planetary Formulas* and *Source Naturals* lines to national prominence. Mark credits Roy Upton and Michael Tierra for his understanding of herbs, while holding them entirely blameless for what he does not yet know. His contributions to this book are based primarily on reviews of current research.

HOW TO USE THIS BOOK

This book contains current research source materials on forty-four (44) different herbs. They are listed alphabetically throughout the book (see the Table of Contents in the beginning for specific listings). Some pages include a simple illustration of the whole herb. Each herb listing contains a reference section, underneath the Herb name, citing the *common name*, *latin name*, *origin*, *part of the plant used*, the *active substances* and the recognized *standard*. Then brief paragraphs follow giving: *Descriptions* of the herb; *Pharmacology*; *The Historical Uses* of the herb, *Active Properties*, the methods by which the herb has been *Processed; Directions* for using the herb; any *Bio-Enhancing Agents*; any *Toxicity, Cautions or Contra-Indications* known to the herb; an *Analysis* of the Standardized extract ; and finally, a detailed listing of the *Scientific References* used to compile the information.

There are two ways that cross reference materials may be accessed: (1) by looking up an alphabetically listed disease or condition in the index (pages 85-95) where a list of herbs indicated for that use is arranged to the right of the condition; or (2) by turning to pages 96-103 where herbs and conditions have been organized into a quick reference chart for easy referral, both are listed alphabetically.

In the back of the book on page 104, there is a list of current manufacturers and distributors of standardized herbal products.

DISCLAIMER

IMPORTANT ! The information contained in this book is intended for educational purposes only. It is not provided to diagnose, prescribe, or treat any disease, illness or injured condition of the body, and the authors, publisher, printer, and distributor accept no responsibility for such use. Those indiviuals suffering from any disease, illness or injury should consult with a physician or health care professional.

AGNUS CASTUS (VITEX)
Chaste Berry

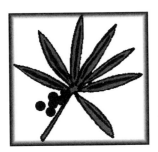

COMMON NAME
Chasteberry Tree, Monk's Pepper, Chaste Tree, Hemp tree, Abraham's balm, Vitex agnus-castus

LATIN NAME
Vitex Agnus-Castus

ORIGIN
Mediterranean area, Israel

PART OF THE PLANT USED
Dried Fruit

ACTIVE SUBSTANCES
Iridoid glycosides, including agnuside, aucubin, and eurostosid; flavonoids including casticin, chryso splenol, and vitexin.

STANDARD
5000 ppm agnuside,
6000 ppm aucubin.

DESCRIPTION
Vitex Agnus-Castus is a deciduous bush or tree, common to southern Europe and the countries of the Mediterranean basin. It is known as the chaste tree for its reputed power to restrain or reduce sexual desire in both women and men. The tree is a form of wild lilac and has similar pink-violet fragrant flowers and arrays of light green pointed leaves. The medicinal part is the berry which is small and hard, similar to a peppercorn. Now, for the first time, this plant is available as a standardized extract.

PHARMACOLOGY
The precise active ingredients are unknown. The berries as well as the leaves contain an aromatic oil with a variety of unique compounds. The iridoid glycosides (monoterpenes), including agnuside, aucubin, and eurostosid are the major unique constituents considered to be medicinally active. The plant is thought to contain a progesterone-like compound. Studies in Germany showed that extracts of Agnus castus stimulated the release of Luteinizing Hormone (LH) and inhibited the release of Follicle Stimulating Hormone (FSH), both progesterone-like effects.

ACTIVE PROPERTIES
Agnus castus has been used since ancient times as a female remedy, controlling and regulating the female reproductive system. It was used to regularize monthly periods and to treat amenorrhea and dysmenorrhea. In addition it was used to help ease menopausal symptoms and the birth process. Modern research and usage have shown that Agnus castus can regulate disturbed female hormonal action, reduce menstrual and menopausal symptoms, especially premenstrual tension, amenorrhea, dysmenorrhea, and endometriosis. One study on premenstrual tension reported that symptoms such as anxiety, nervous tension, insomnia, and mood changes were the most reduced after taking dried Agnus castus tablets.

PROCESSING
The fruit of the chasteberry tree is wild-harvested from countries in the Mediterranean area, mainly from Israel. Extraction is exhaustive using only alcohol/wa-

HISTORICAL USES

- Amenorrhea
- Dysmenorrhea
- Menopause
- Premenstrual tension, anxiety, nervous tension insomnia, mood changes
- Endometriosis
- Birth process
- Irregular menstrual cycles

AGNUS CASTUS (VITEX)
Chaste Berry

ter (no organic solvents). The extract is spray dried on a special carrier to produce a stable powder which is then standardized.

DIRECTIONS FOR USE
400 mg/day standardized extract, equivalent to 2.0 gm/day of dried berries.

TOXICITY, CAUTIONS & CONTRA-INDICATIONS
No known toxicity.

SCIENTIFIC REFERENCES
• Jochle, W. (1974) Menses-inducing Drugs: Their role in antique, medieval, and renaissance gynaecology and birth control. Contraception. 10:425.
• Hansel, R. and Winde, E. (1959) Constituents of the Verbenacae 2 Agnuside, a new glycoside from Vitex agnus castus. L. Arzneimittel. Forschung. 9:180-190.
• Wollenweber, E. and Mann, K. (1983) Flavonols from the fruits of Vitex agnus-castus. Planta Medica. 48:126-127.
• Gomas, C.S. et al. (1978) Flavonoids and Iridoids from VItex agnus castus. Planta Medica 33:277.
• Haller, J. (1958) Animal experimentation with the Lipschutz technics on the activity of a phytohormone on gonadotropin function. Geburtschilfe Frauenheilkund. 18:1347.
• Stewart, A. (1987) Gerard Agnus castus in Premenstrual Tension, available from Gerard House Ltd. Bournemouth, England.

ANALYSIS

Product:	*Vitex Agnus castus* berries	
Type:	Standardized extract	
Quality:	Traditional, wild-harvested	
	Specification	Result
Agnuside (HPLC)	.5%	.50%
Aucubin (HPLC)		.40%
Loss on drying:	<7%	2.26%
Color		conforms
pH:	4.5-5.5	4.93
Ash:	<7%	5.82%
Mesh size		<80
Bulk density:loose/packed		.46/.56 g /ml
Heavy Metals		conforms
Pestiside residues		conforms
Microbiology total count per gr	1000	conforms
E. coli	<10	conforms
Coliforms	<30	conforms
Staph. aureus	<10	conforms
salmonella	neg	conforms
yeasts and moulds	<20	conforms

ARTICHOKE
(Globe)

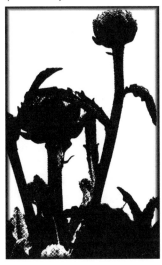

COMMON NAME
Artichoke, Globe artichoke
LATIN NAME
Cynara scolymus
ORIGIN
Northern United States
and Europe
PART OF THE PLANT USED
Flower heads, Leaves, Root
ACTIVE SUBSTANCES
Cynarin, sesquiterpene lactones, Flavonoids scolymoside, inulin, cynaropictin, taraxasterol
STANDARD
(1) 15% caffeylquinic acid
(chlorogenic acid)
(2) 2-5% cynarin

DESCRIPTION
The flower head of the globe artichoke is used as a common food. The artichoke head, leaves and root contain several active components important for digestion and for liver, kidney and gall bladder complaints. Traditional uses have included sluggish liver, poor digestion and atherosclerosis.

PHARMACOLOGY
Artichokes contain cynarin and scolymoside which have been shown to stimulate bile secretion. Cynarin also has been reported to lower cholesterol and triglyceride levels. Artichoke also contains some diuretic activities and has been used for kidney diseases and proteinuria.

DIRECTIONS FOR USE
200 mg. / day herbal extract

BIO-ENHANCING AGENTS
Turmeric, Milk Thistle, Licorice Root

TOXICITY, CAUTIONS & CONTRAINDICATIONS
No known toxicity.

PROCESSING
Hydroalcoholic extract

SCIENTIFIC REFERENCES
• Mowrey, D. (1988) Guaranteed Potency Herbs. Next Generation Herbal Medicine. Lehi, UT: Cormorant Books

HISTORICAL USES

- sluggish liver, increase bile secretion;
- poor digestion;
- atherosclerosis;
- elevated triglycerides, elevated cholesterol;
- diuretic, kidney diseases, proteinuria

ANALYSIS

(1) 15% caffeylquinic acid

Determination:	Results
Spectrophotometric Contents:	15.82%
of caffeylquinic acids calculated as chlorogenic acid	
Character:	complies
Appearance:	yellow-brown powder
TLC ID	complies
pH:(c=1, water)	5.5
Sulfated Ash:	13.8%
Water (K. Fischer)	1.71%
Heavy metals	<100.0 ppm
Total Residual Organic Solvents	0.005%
Ethanol	<0.005%
Total amount of other solvents	0.005%

(2) 5% Cynarin

Determination:	Results
Moisture content	4%
Mesh size	100 mesh
Mfg. Standard	5% Cynarin min.
Extraction Ratio	30:1
preservative	none
pH	4.5-5.5
Solubility	water soluble
Color	brown
Odor	Characteristic
Taste	Characteristic
Plate count	pass

ASTRAGALUS

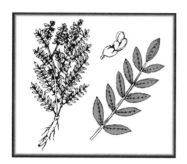

COMMON NAME
Milk Vetch, Locoweed, Yellow Vetch, Poison Vetch, Chinese Astragalus, Huang Ch'i

LATIN NAME
Astragalus membranaceus

ORIGIN
China, Taiwan, Korea

PART OF PLANT USED
Roots

ACTIVE SUBSTANCES
Isoflavones, triterpenoid saponins including astragalosides I to VIII, astramembrannins, and soya-sapogenols, polysaccharides, choline, betaine, kumatakenin

STANDARD
0.4% minimum 4'-Hydroxy-3'-methoxyisoflavone 7-sug

DESCRIPTION
Chinese Astragalus, or "Huang Ch'i" belongs to the group of Vetches and the family of peas. The plant is known as the milk vetch. Astragalus is a mild restorative and preventive plant.

PHARMACOLOGY/ PHYSIOLOGY
Astragalus contains a unique isoflavone, termed 4' hydroxy-3'-methoxyisoflavone 7-sug which has some pharmacological activities on digestion. Other ingredients of Astragalus include the triterpenoid saponins (Astragalosides, astramem-brannins) which are analogous to the animal steroid hormones. Also important in Astragalus are the numerous polysaccharides which have shown in pharmacological experiments to enhance the activity of the immune system, particularly NK and T cell function, and increased interferon production.

ACTIVE PROPERTIES/ INDICATIONS
Astragalus, one of the most important Oriental tonic and health-promoting medicinal plants, has been classically used in the Orient to strengthen the Wei Ch'i or defensive energy and to "warm" the exterior. Thus Astragalus is widely used to increase resistance to disease and infections, to restore depressed immunity, to treat hepatitis, AIDS, and other viral conditions, and to treat peripheral vascular diseases and restore peripheral circulation. Recent research has revealed possible uses for myasthenia gravis, immune depletion in cancer patients, ARC, influenza and other viral infections, hypertension, and ischemia.

DIRECTIONS FOR USE
4 gm./day root or 1 gm/day of extract

PROCESSING
Similar to traditional methods: the roots are sun-dried, graded, and sliced. Water/alcohol extraction at low temperature, followed by drying to create a stable free-flowing powder.

HISTORICAL USES

- Oriental tonic and health promoter
- Increase resistance to disease and infections
- Restore depressed immunity
- To treat peripheral vascular disease, hypertension, ischemia.
- To restore peripheral circulation
- For myasthenia gravis
- For immune depletion in cancer patients
- To boost the immune system in ARC, influenza, and other viral conditions

ASTRAGALUS

TOXICITY, CAUTIONS & CONTRA-INDICATIONS

No known toxicity.

SCIENTIFIC REFERENCES

• Kitagawa, I., et al. (1983) Saponin and Sapogenin. 35. Chemical Constituents of Astragali radix, the root of Astragalus membranaceous 2, Astragolosides 1,2, and 4, Acetylastragaloside 1, and Isoastragalosides 1 and 2. Chem. Pharm. Bull. 31:698-708.

• Wang, Z.X., et al. (1983) Studies on the chemical constituents of astragalus (Astragalus membranaceous). Chung Tsao Yao 14:97-99.

• Hikino, H., et al. (1976) Validity of Oriental Medicines. 2. Hypotensive Principle of Astragalus and Hedysarum Roots. Planta Medica 30:297.

• Hou, Y. et al. (1981) Effect of Radix Astragali Seu Hedysari on the Interferon System. Chin. Med. J. 94:35-40.

• Mingxing, Sh. et al. (1982) Therapeutic effect of Astragalus in treating chronic active hepatitis and the changes in immune functions. J. of Chinese People's Liberation Army 7:242-4.

• Chen, K. (1981) Certain progress in the treatment of coronary heart disease with traditional medicinal plants. Amer. J. Chinese Med. (:193-196.

• Kou, W. et al. (1983). Clinical effect of "Yi gi Huo Xue" medicinal herbs in Acute Myocardial Infarction: a randomized controlled study. Chinese J. Integr. Tradit. West. Med. 3:146-148.

• Lim, D. Y. (1979) A study on the hypotensive action of Astragali Radix water extract in the rabbit. Yakhak Hoe Chi. 23:69-80.

ANALYSIS

Product:	*Astragalus membranaceous* root
Color:	Light, brown powder
Flavor:	Sweet with bitter undertones
Standardization:	
4'-Hydroxy-3'-methoxyisoflavone 7-sug	(min. .4%) .53%
pH	6.03
Total Ash	4.93%
Loss on drying: (vacuum at 100-105°C for 3 hours)	7.62%
Mesh size:	conforms
Bulk density:	.65/.72
Heavy metals:	conforms
Pesticides:	<0.05
Microbiology: total count	200/g
e.coli	<10
Coliform	<10
S. Aureus	<10
Salmonella	neg
yeasts & molds	<10

BILBERRY

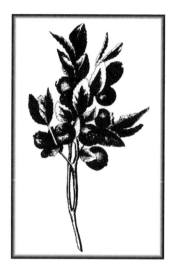

COMMON NAME
Bilberry, Huckleberry,
Whortleberry
LATIN NAME
Vaccinium myrtillus L.
ORIGIN
Europe (wild)
PART OF THE PLANT USED
Fresh fruit
ACTIVE SUBSTANCES
anthocyanosides, flavonoids
STANDARD
25 % anthocyanosides calcu-
lated as anthocyanidins

DESCRIPTION
Bilberry is a perennial shrub native to Northern Europe, Northern
America, and Canada. The Bilberry plant produces a fruit similar
to the American blueberry, but
containing higher quantities of
constituents useful for visual acuity and night blindness.

PHARMACOLOGY
Bilberry is rich in anthocyanosides. Over 15 different
anthocyanosides have been found
in Bilberry. Anthocyanosides help
to maintain the integrity of capillaries and to stabilize collagen.
Anthocyanosides are also potent
antioxidants. Numerous clinical
studies have shown that Bilberry
is effective in the treatment of circulation disorders, varicose veins,
and other venous and arterial disorders. The anthocyanosides protect veins and arteries by stabiliz-
ing the phospholipids of the endothelial cells, and by increasing
the synthesis of collagen and mucopolysaccharides which give the
arterial walls their structural integrity. Antho-cyanosides also prevent the aggregation and adherence of platelets to endothelial
surfaces. Studies have also shown
that Bilberry can act as a coadjutant
in heme-ralopy and diabetic
retinopathy and can stimulate
rhodopsin production.

PROCESSING
Extraction with hydromethanolic
solution.

DIRECTIONS FOR USE
3each of -80 mg. capsules/day

HISTORICAL USES

Ophthalmology:
• Myopia
• Retinal disturbances
• Eye strain / visual acuity
• Dark adaptation
• Day and night blindness
• Pigmentary retinitis
• Diabetic-induced cataracts.

Vascular Disorders:
• Blood purpuras
• Varicose veins
• Varices
• Anti-coagulating problems
• Capillary fragility and hyper-permeability
• Phlebitis
• Hypertension
• Advanced diabetic vascular complications
• Arteriosclerosis
• Hemorrhages
• Bleeding gums
• Kidney hematuria
• CNS vascular disorders.

BILBERRY

TOXICITY, CAUTIONS & CONTRAINDICATIONS

No known toxicity.

SCIENTIFIC REFERENCES

• Jonadet, M. et al. (1983) Anthocyanosides extracted from Vitis vinifera, Vaccinium myrtillus, and Pinus maritimus. I. Elastase-inhibiting activities in vitro. II. Compared angiopro-tective activities in vivo. J. Pharm. Belg. 38:41-46.

• Detre, A. et al. (1986) Studies on vascular permeability in hypertension: action of anthocyan-osides. Clin. Physiol. Biochem. 4:143-9.

• Ronziere, M.C. et al. (1981) Influence of some flavonoids on reticulation of collagen fibrils in vitro. Biochem Pharmacol. 30:1771-6.

• Mian, E. et al. (1977) Anthocyanosides and the walls of the microvessels: further aspects of the mechanism of action of their protective effect in syndromes due to abnormal capillary fragility. Minerva Med. 68:3565-81.

• Lietti, A. and Forni, G. (1976) Studies on Vaccinium myrtillus anthocyanosides. I. Vasoprotective and anti-inflammatory activity. Arzneim Forsch. 26:829-32.

• Bottecchia, D. et al. (1987) Preliminary report on the inhibitory effect of Vaccinium myrtillus anthocyanosides on platelet aggregation and clot retraction. Fitoterapia 48:3-8.

• Bettini, V. et al. (1984) Effects of Vaccinium myrtillus anthocyanosides on vascular smooth muscle. Fitoterapia 55:265-72.

ANALYSIS

Product:	*Vaccinium myrtillus L.* fruit
Type:	Standardized extract
Quality:	wild-crafted
Color:	dark, red-violet powder
Standardization:	25 % anthocyanosides (anthocyanidins)
Solubility in chloroform	insoluble
Solubility in acetone	insoluble
Sulfated ash:	0.5 %
Water (K. Fischer)	3.83%
Heavy metals:	<40 ppm
Total residual organic solvents	0.435 %
Total amount other solvents	.005%
Total residual aerobic microbial count:	< 1000 cfu/g
Fungi	<100 cfu/g
S. aureus, Salmonella, E. coli, P. aeruginosa	absent

BROCCOLI CRUCIFEROUS EXTRACT

DESCRIPTION

Broccoli (Brassica oleracea Botrytis cymosa) is a dark green vegetable in the cruciferous family. It is rich in fiber, provitamin A carotenoids, vitamin C and vitamin K. Fresh broccoli is available throughout the year, with the peak season from January through March. This is a cruciferous vegetable extract, standardized for sulforaphane.

PHARMACOLOGY

Cruciferous vegetables apparently can reduce the risk of cancer by inducing extra protection of the enzymes involved in detoxifying carcinogens and flushing them out of the body. The phase II enzymes, including quinone reductase and glutathione S-tranferase, are particularly active. Sulforaphane is a major and very potent phase II enzyme inducer. Sulforaphane, along with other cancer-protective isothiocyanates, does not induce damaging phase I enzymes. Besides protecting against the risk of cancer occuring, sulforaphane appears to reduce the severity of cancers that do occur.

Estrogen is formed from estradiol, and can take either a safe, relatively inert form, 2-hydroxylated, or a dangerously reactive form that has been associated with breast cancers and increased risk of breast cancer, 16-hydroxylated estrogen. Indoles, particularly indole-3-carbinol, induce protection of the safe, rather than the dangerously reactive, form of estrogen. 2-hydroxylated estrogen is also induced by vigorous exercise (at least 2, and preferably 4 hours per week), and a major study released in September 1994 showed a strong correlation with reduced cancer risk. Broccoli may have other antioxidant activities due to its carotenoid, phenolic and anthocyanin constituents.

ACTIVE PROPERTIES

Key nutritional constituents are fiber, provitamin A carotenoids, vitamin C and vitamin K. Isothiocyanates are a class of compounds recently identified at Johns Hopkins University as being one key to the anticancer properties of cruciferous vegetables. The most active isothiocyanate is sulforaphane.

Fresh, commercial broccoli has widely varying amounts of isothiocyanates and sulforaphane, depending on the plant strain, growing methods and time of harvesting. Also, the absorption and utilization of these compounds can be hampered by poor preparation or digestion. Therefore, extracts of broccoli and other cruciferous vegetables that concentrate

HISTORICAL USES

- Broccoli helps prevent stomach and colon cancer, as do other members of the cruciferous family.

- It is also a good dietary source of fiber, provitamin A carotenoids, vitamin C and vitamin K.

COMMON NAME
Broccoli, Kale and Radish
LATIN NAME
Brassica oleracea Botrytis cymosa (Broccoli)
Brassica oleracea var. acephala (Kale)
Raphanus sativus (Radish)
ORIGIN
United States
PART OF THE PLANT USED
Stem and flower buds
ACTIVE SUBSTANCES
Sulforaphane, indole-3-carbinol
STANDARD
>=40 mg Sulforaphane / 100 g

BROCCOLI CRUCIFEROUS EXTRACT

isothiocyanates and sulforaphane by factors of from 133:1 to 400:1 have been developed, to provide enhanced protection. Indoles are another key to anticancer activity. Dr. H. Leon Bradlow of the Strang-Cornell Cancer Research Laboratory in New York has isolated a crucial one, indole-3-carbinol, from broccoli.

DIRECTIONS FOR USE
250 mg of a 400:1 extract at 0.4 mg / g sulforaphane is equivalent to one serving (100 grams) of fresh commercial broccoli.

TOXICITY, CAUTIONS & CONTRAINDICATIONS
No known toxicity.

SCIENTIFIC REFERENCES

• Zhang, Y., Talalay, P., Cho, C. G., & Posner, G.H., A major inducer of anticarcinogenic protective enzymes from broccoli: Isolation and elucidation of structure, Proc. Natl. Acad. Sci. USA, vol. 89, pp.2399-2403, March 1992.
• Prochaska, H.J., Santamaria, A.B., & Talalay, P., Rapid detection of inducers of enzymes that protect against cancer, Proc. Natl. Acad. Sci. USA, vol. 89, pp.2394-2398, March 1992.
• Cancer Research (Suppl.), vol. 52, pg.2085, 1992.
• J. Natl. Cancer Inst., vol. 83, pg. 541, 1991.
• Bernstein, L., [moderate but regular physical activity reduces risk of premenopausal breast cancer] J. Natl. Cancer Insti., Sept.21, 1994.

ANALYSIS

Product Name:	Broccoli / Cruciferous 40 Extract
Genus:	Brassica oleracea Botrytis cymosa (Broccoli)
	Brassica oleracea var. acephala (Kale)
	Raphanus sativus (Radish)
Excipients:	Cellulose
Solvent for Extraction:	Hydro-Alcohol
Particle Size:	95% through 80 mesh screen
Color:	green
Odor:	Strong broccoli smell
Taste:	Strong broccoli taste
Standardization: (by HPLC)	>=40 mg Sulforaphane / 100 g
Loss on drying:	<5%
Bulk / Density:	0.29 g / cc
Aerobic Plate:	<10,000 cfu / g
E. coli	Neg. (<10 cfu / g)
Coliform	Neg. (<10 cfu / g)
Yeast	<100 cfu / g
Mold	<100 cfu / g
Salmonella	Negative

BUTCHER'S BROOM

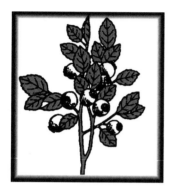

DESCRIPTION
Butcher's Broom is an evergreen shrub native to the Mediterranean region and a member of the Lily family. The plant derives its name from the use of the stiff twigs as brushes by butchers for their cutting blocks. The rhizome of this plant has been used since the ancient times of the Greeks for many circulatory disorders. Greek Doctors treated swelling and varicose veins with Butcher's Broom.

PHARMACOLOGY
Butcher's Broom contains saponin glycosides called rusco-genins. Research has shown that these ruscogenins possess vasoconstrictive and anti-inflammatory properties. These active ingredients reduce the fragility and permeability of capillaries and constrict the veins. These plant saponin glycosides are the starter compounds for important steroid compounds in the human body.

ACTIVE PROPERTIES
Butcher's broom extract was found to possess vasoconstrictive and anti-inflammatory properties. The herb is used in European medicine for venous circulatory disorders and hemorrhoidal problems. Many European women use Butcher's Broom to reduce capillary fragility and to help prevent edema in the legs after standing all day. Others have used the herb for varicose veins, particularly during pregnancy.

PROCESSING
Extraction with hydroalcoholic solution.

DIRECTIONS FOR USE
150 mg./day internal. Can be used externally as poultice, ointment or suppository.

BIO-ENHANCING AGENTS
Bilberry, centella, ginkgo biloba, ginger root, horse chestnut.

COMMON NAME
Butcher's Broom
LATIN NAME
Ruscus aculeatus L.
ORIGIN
Europe (wild)
PART OF PLANT USED
Rhizome
ACTIVE SUBSTANCES
Ruscogenins
(saponin glycosides)
STANDARD
10% ruscogenins from whole Butcher's Broom

HISTORICAL USES

- **Proctology**: hemorrhoids, proctitis, pruritus ani (anal itching), anal fissures

- **Phlebology:** varicose veins, varices, chilblains, "heavy legs" , surface veins, post-thrombotic syndrome, venous circulatory disorders

- **Ophthalmology:** diabetic retinopathy, retinal hemorrhages

- **Gynecology:** menstrual problems, troubles with taking estrogens, cramps of pregnancy, varicose veins of pregnancy

BUTCHER'S BROOM

TOXICITY, CAUTIONS & CONTRA-INDICATIONS

Occasional allergy-induced nausea or gastritis.

SCIENTIFIC REFERENCES

• Capra, C. (1972) Studio farmacologico e tossicologico di componenti del ruscus aculeatus L. Fitoterapia. 43:99.

• Chabanon, R. (1976) Experimentation du Proctolog dans les hemorroides et les fissures anales. Gaz. Med. De France. 83:3013.

• Mowrey, D. (1990) Guaranteed Potency Herbs. A Compilation of writings on the subject.

• Weiner, M. (1990) Weiner's Herbal. Mill Valley: Quantum Books.

• Tyler, V.E. et al.(1988) Pharma-cognosy, 9th Ed. Philadelphia, PA: Lea & Febiger.

ANALYSIS

Determination	Results
Spectrophotometric Contents of sapponins calculated as ruscogenins	10.0%
Appearance	Light Brown powder
Characteristics	complies
TLC ID	complies
pH (c=5, alcohol [60% v/v])	5.4
Loss on drying (T=105C, t=3h)	4.56
Sulfated Ash	5.96%
Heavy Metals	complies
Total residual organic solvents	0.56%
Ethanol	.415%
Methanol	0.05%
Isopropanol	0.02%
Cyclohexane	0.075 ppm
Other solvents	<50.0 ppm
Total Aerobic	<1000.0cfu/g
fungi	<100.0 cfu/g
Staph. aureus, salmonella	absent
E. coli	absent

CASCARA SAGRADA

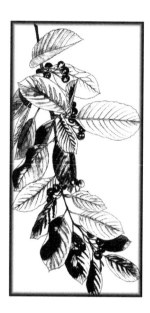

COMMON NAME
Cascara sagrada, shittim, wahoo

LATIN NAME
Rhamnus purshiana

ORIGIN
Pacific Northwest

PART OF PLANT USED
Dried Bark

ACTIVE SUBSTANCES
Hydroxy anthracene derivatives (HAD)

STANDARD
20-30% Hydroxy anthracene derivatives (HAD)

DESCRIPTION

Cascara sagrada, "sacred bark" in Spanish, is a deciduous shrub or small tree from the buckthorn family with a distinctive reddish gray bark. The name dates back to the seventeenth century when the American Indians introduced the Spanish and Mexican explorers to the usefulness of the bark for constipation and upset stomach. The bark was first marketed to the medical community in 1877 when the pharmaceutical company of Parke-Davis introduced a bitter emetic fluid extract. In 1890 the plant was officially listed in the U.S. Pharmacopoea.

PHARMACOLOGY

Free anthraquinone and its sugar derivative, hydroxyanthracene derivative (HAD) are the active ingredients responsible for the laxative effect. These active substances cause an increased peristalsis locally in the large intestine and also act at a distance by circulating in the bloodstream and stimulating a nerve center to trigger a laxative effect.

ACTIVE PROPERTIES

Cascara is perhaps the safest and most certain laxative available and can be used to restore tone to the colon and thereby overcome laxative dependence in the elderly. The herb is safe and effective for detoxifying and cleansing programs, as opposed to the harsher laxatives, such as senna. Cascara is also an effective liver tonic in small doses: hepatitis, gall stones, etc. Cascara can be used as an effective chelating agent to prevent the occurrence of calcium-based urinary stones.

PROCESSING

The bark is stripped from the trees in spring and fall and then dried to render it more acceptable to the digestive system and then pulverized.

DIRECTIONS FOR USE

50-100 mg of 25% HAD depending on degree of constipation. Elderly and small children should use 1/4 to 1/2 the normal dosage.

BIO-ENHANCING AGENTS

As a laxative: Butternut Root Bark, Frangula, Licorice Root, Irish Moss; As a liver tonic: Dandelion, Milk Thistle, Shisandra, Licorice Root, Wild Yam.

HISTORICAL USES

- Laxative
- Cathartic
- Purgative
- Liver tonic
- Cholagogue
- Antibacterial Agent
- Chelating Agent

CASCARA SAGRADA

TOXICITY, CAUTIONS & CONTRA-INDICATIONS

No toxicity at recommended dosages. Use only as directed. Takes from six to eight hours to produce stool. Cathartic effect at very high doses. Should not be used by nursing mothers since the laxative effect will be transmitted to their infants. Should not be used by people suffering from ulcers or irritable bowel syndrome.

SCIENTIFIC REFERENCES

• Mowrey, D. (1990) Guaranteed Potency Herbs. A Compilation of writings on the subject.

ANALYSIS

Determination	Results
Spectrophotometric Contents of dihydroxyanthracenic etherosides calculated as cascaroside A	20.4%
Spectrophotometric Contents of cascarosides on the total amount of dihydroxyanthracenic etherosides	73.0%
Characteristics	brown powder with a bitter taste
TLC ID	complies
pH (c=5, alcohol [50% v/v])	5.5
Loss on drying (T=110C, p=5mmHg, t=16h)	0.6%
Sulfated Ash	4.6%
Heavy Metals	complies ppm
Total residual organic solvents	0.56%
Total Aerobic	<40.0cfu/g
fungi	<100.0 cfu/g
Staph. aureus, salmonella	absent
E. coli	absent

CHAMOMILE

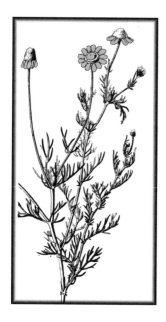

COMMON NAME
German Chamomile,
Roman Chamomile

LATIN NAME
Matricaria chamomilla
Matricaria recutita
Chamaemelum nobile

ORIGIN
Southern Europe

PART OF PLANT USED
Fresh flowers

ACTIVE SUBSTANCES
Flavonoids (Apigenine
and luteoline), Bisabolols,
en-indicycloether, matricine,
chamazulene, and essential
oils

STANDARD
1.2% Apigenin and
0.5 % essential oil.
Whole plant material.

DESCRIPTION
Chamomile has been described by the Germans as *"Alles zutraut"*, meaning "capable of anything" because of the belief that chamomile can cure almost anything. Teas, ointments, lotions, extracts, and inhalations have been made and used for both medicinal and cosmetic purposes.

PHARMACOLOGY
The active ingredients are found in the essential volatile oil derived from the flowers. Extracts of the plant or the essential oil have been used as anti-inflam-matories, as anti-spasmodics, and as anti-infectives. Standardized chamomile with at least 1% apigenin and 0.5% essential oil are guarantees that the extract contains all important constituents. Bisabolols, enindicyclo-ether, and the flavonoids such as apiginine and luteoline have been found to be necessary for chamomile's anti-inflammatory, calming, mildly sedative, and anti-spasmodic effects. Azulene, chamazuline, bisabolol, and matricine are the more anti-inflammatory constituents. Azulene has been shown to inhibit histamine release and to block the effect of serotonin. All the major active principles of chamomile are necessary to get optimal effects.

ACTIVE PROPERTIES
Chamomile is frequently used as a mild sedative, to calm the nerves reduce anxiety, and induce a state of pleasant relaxation without disrupting normal function or interfering with motor coordination. Chamomile is also used as a carminative, calming upset stomachs, and easing digestion. Chamomile's effectiveness is also due to its anti-inflammatory properties, soothing ulcers and reducing

HISTORICAL USES

Folklore:
- Anodyne, analgesic, antiseptic, antiphlogistic, antispasmodic, calmative, sedative, diaphoretic, tonic, vulnerary

Research/Clinical:
Internal:
- Calming, slightly sedative on nerves;
- Induces relaxation
- Uterine tonic (good for menstrual cramps)
- Prevent and treat ulcers and other forms of gastrointestinal distress including indigestion, heartburn, gastritis, diverticulitis, and flatulence
- Treat and prevent anxiety, insomnia, nervousness, restlessness, stress.

External:
- Antiseptic, antibiotic, vulnerary for burns, sores, chapped skin, dryness, cuts, abrasions, eczema, allergic exanthemas, dermatitis, inflammation, infections, tumors, and wounds
- Stomatology: Mouthwash for gingivitis, ulcerative stomatitis, paradentosis, pharyngitis, esophagitis, sequelae of sinusitis.

CHAMOMILE

gastritis and other mucous membrane inflammations. One of the most popular uses for chamomile has been in creams and lotions for the skin. Treatment with chamomile helps burns, wounds, infections ,acne, etc. to heal more rapidly. Chamomile has good anti-bacterial action, particularly against staph and strep toxins, as well as anti-fungal action against *Candida albicans.*

PROCESSING
The flowers are harvested when the petals begin to turn back on the disk

DIRECTIONS FOR USE
1-4 of 400 mg. capsules daily, depending on level of nervousness or anxiety.

BIO-ENHANCING AGENTS
Externally: Aloe Vera.
Internally: Passion Flower, Goldenseal, Yellow Dock, Kelp, Valerian Root, Peppermint, Vitamin B Complex, Vitamin C, Vitamin A.

TOXICITY, CAUTIONS & CONTRA-INDICATIONS
No toxicity. Rare cases of allergic reactions in persons with severe hypersensitivity to ragweed pollen. Avoid contact with eyes. Depressant in high doses.

SCIENTIFIC REFERENCES
• Mowrey, D. (1990) Guaranteed Potency Herbs. A Compilation of writings on the subject.
• Mowrey, D. (19) The Scientific Validation of Herbal Medicine.
• Kowalchik, C. and Hylton, W., eds. (1987) Rodale's Illustrated Encyclopedia of Herbs. Emmaus, Pennsylvania: Rodale Press.

ANALYSIS

Determination	Results
HPLC Contents	1.50%
of total apigenin	
Characteristics	yellow-brown hygroscopic amorphous powder
Solubility in water(c=2)	clear/opalescent solution
in alcohol (50% v/v)(c=2)	clear/opalescent solution
TLC ID	complies
pH (c=1, water)	4.9
Sulfated Ash	6.3%
Water (K. Fischer)	1.8%
Heavy Metals	complies
Total residual organic solvents	0.07%
Ethanol	0.07%
total amount other solvents	<0.005%
Total Aerobic	<1000 cfu/g
fungi	<100 cfu/g
Staph. aureus, salmonella	absent
E. coli	absent

DEVIL'S CLAW

DESCRIPTION

Devil's Claw derives its name from its large hooked, claw-like fruit which has been known to harm and trap livestock grazing nearby. The tuber is used medicinally and has become a primary treatment for arthritis and rheumatism. In the Kalahari Desert and Namibian steppes, the root is also used as a treatment for indigestion and other gastro-intestinal problems in the same manner as Western bitters are used. Devil's claw is also used externally as an ointment to treat skin rashes, wounds, etc.

PHARMACOLOGY

Two components of the plant, harpogoside and beta sitosterol have anti-inflammatory properties. Whole Devil's Claw however was found to be superior to isolated harpogoside. Devil's Claw also possesses a bitter value of 6,000 equivalent to gentian root, the main western bitter.

ACTIVE PROPERTIES

Devil's Claw has been used in Africa and German medical clinics for liver, gall bladder, and kidney ailments, lymphatic system toxicity, diabetes, nervous malaise, respiratory ailments, blood diseases, and indigestion. Most clinical studies have shown that this plant has strong anti-inflammatory properties and is extremely helpful for sufferers of arthritis and inflammatory diseases. Devil's claw was reported helpful to reduce swelling relieve pain, improve motility in the joints, and improved feeling of well-being. The British Herbal Pharmacopoea recognizes Devil's Claw as having anti-inflammatory, anti-rheumatic, analgesic, sedative, and diuretic properties. In addition Devil's Claw has proved effective in treating such complaints as dyspepsia and conditions relating to the proper functioning of bile salts, the gallbladder, and the enterohepatic circuit.

COMMON NAME
Devil's Claw
LATIN NAME
Harpogophytum procumbens
ORIGIN
Africa,
particularly South Africa
PART OF THE PLANT USED
tuber, roots
ACTIVE SUBSTANCES
Iridoid glycosides (harpogoside, harpagide, and procumbine), sugars, gum resin, Beta-sitosterol
STANDARD
5% harpogosides,
whole plant material

HISTORICAL USES

- Arthritis, gout, rheumatism, gout, spondylosis-induced lower back pain
- Inflammation, analgesic, sedative, anti-spasmodic
- Relieve pain and swelling
- Edema, water retention
- Indigestion, upset stomach, dyspepsia, bile salt problems
- Liver, gallbladder, and kidney ailments
- Elevated blood sugar
- Sluggish immune systems

DEVIL'S CLAW

PROCESSING
Dry, aqueous extract

DIRECTIONS FOR USE
100 mg/day of 5% standardized
extract

BIO-ENHANCING AGENTS
Oregon grape root, black cohosh,
guaiacum, ginger root.

**TOXICITY, CAUTIONS &
CONTRA-INDICATIONS**
Side effects are rare. Devil's Claw
should be avoided during pregnancy as it has been suggested to
stimulate uterine muscle. Devil's
Claw has extremely low toxicity
with the LD50 established at 34
mg./kg. and 220 mg./kg.

SCIENTIFIC REFERENCES
• Mowrey, D. (1990) Guaranteed Potency
Herbs. A Compilation of writings on the
subject.
• Mowrey, D. (1986) The Scientific Vali-
dation of Herbal Medicine. Cormorant
Books.

ANALYSIS

Product:	Devil's claw, *Harpogophytum procumbens*
Type	Standardized extract
Quality	traditional
Color	light brown powder
Standardization	>50% Glycoiridoids calculated as Harpogoside
Loss on drying	<8.0%
pH (10% solution)	from 5 to 6
Ash	<20%(DAB-10)
Heavy Metals	No more than 60 ppm
Microbiological Specifications	absent
Storage	Store sealed in a cool dry place

17

DONG QUAI
Chinese Angelica

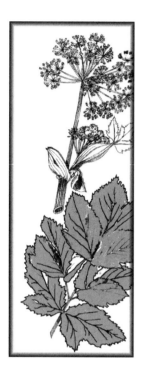

COMMON NAME
Chinese Angelica
Dong Quai
LATIN NAME
Angelica sinensis
A. polymorpha, A. acutiloba
ORIGIN
Asia, primarily China, Korea, Japan.
PART OF THE PLANT USED
dried root
ACTIVE SUBSTANCES
ligustilide, butyl phthalide, butylene phthalide, ferulic acid, polysaccharides
STANDARD
8000 ppm to 11000 ppm of ligustilide

DESCRIPTION
Chinese Angelica, "Dong Quai" is the most important female tonic remedy in Chinese medicine. It is used for debility and poor vitality, convalescence and tiredness in women as well as all kinds of gynecological, menstrual, or menopausal symptoms. Dong Quai is the Chinese name of the root of the plant *Angelica sinensis* belonging to the family Umbelli-feraceae. It is related to the European Angelica but its medicinal actions are more potent. The plant is a tall umbelliferous plant with branched celery-like leaved and a tall umbel of white-green flowers.

PHARMACOLOGY
Ligustilide, butylene phthalide and butyl phthalide are found in the volatile aromatic oil while ferulic acid and various polysaccharides are found in the non-aromatic fractions. Dong Quai has an immediate and stimulating effect on the uterus, especially during pregnancy or delivery. It has been clinically observed to strengthen and normalize uterine contractions. These effects are thought to be due to components of the volatile oil, particularly ligustilide. Symptoms such as menstrual pain and irregularities, habitual abortion, chills in hands and feet, anemia and in some cases sterility have also responded well to Dong Quai. Animal and human studies have shown that Dong Quai also improves peripheral circulation and reduces blood viscosity. The research suggests that both ferulic acid and ligustilide are responsible, preventing spasms, relaxing vessels, and reducing blood clotting in peripheral vessels.

ACTIVE PROPERTIES
Dong Quai has been used as the main female tonic in the Orient while ginseng has been the more traditional male adaptogen. Dong Quai is used to provide energy, vitality, and resistance to disease. It regulated female hormones, in the treatment of most menstrual and menopausal problems and in pregnancy and delivery. It is a blood tonic, promoting its production and circulation. It is therefore used in treating anemia, boils, headache, venous problems, low immunity, and problems of peripheral blood flow.

HISTORICAL USES

- Menstrual symptoms (amenorrhea, dysmenorrhea, PMS)
- Uterine tonic (good for menstrual cramps)
- Menopausal symptoms
- Anemia
- Low immunity
- Tiredness, poor vitality
- Debility
- Convalescence in women
- Poor peripheral blood flow (intermittent claudication)
- Lowers blood pressure
- Atherosclerosis, high cholesterol
- Relieves pain and swelling
- Liver tonic, protects liver against toxins, stimulates liver metabolism
- Anti-inflammatory, analgesic, sedative, anti-spasmodic, immuno-stimulating

DONG QUAI
Chinese Angelica

PROCESSING

Seeds are planted in autumn. The plant is carefully tended for three years before the roots are ready for harvest. The Dong Quai is dried and selected according to required standards, graded for size of root, strength of taste, growing location and other factors. All raw material is subject to careful checking and analysis in laboratories. Extraction is exhaustive, using a special method to extract all the active ingredients. Only water/alcohol is used similar to traditional methods. No organic solvents are used. The extract is spray dried without carriers to produce a stable pure powder extract which is then standardized. Analysis is done by HPLC of ligustilide content to ensure that the raw material is of the correct identity, variety and good quality.

DIRECTIONS FOR USE

200 mg. standardized extract 3 times daily

BIO-ENHANCING AGENTS:

Licorice root, black cohosh, red raspberry, peony, rehmannia, ginger root, wild yam.

TOXICITY, CAUTIONS & CONTRA-INDICATIONS

No toxicity. Side effects are extremely rare. Rare cases of pyrogenia but requiring no need of treatment. People with gastro-intestinal disease may experience diarrhea. Avoid in case of hemorrhagic disease, hypermenorrhea, first three months of pregnancy, spontaneous abortion, and during severe flu.

SCIENTIFIC REFERENCES

• Mowrey, D. (1990) Guaranteed Potency Herbs. A Compilation of writings on the subject.
• Mowrey, D. (1986) The Scientific Validation of Herbal Medicine. Cormorant Books.
• Teeguarden, R. (1984) Chinese Tonic Herbs. Japan Publications Inc., NY and Tokyo.
• Yaozu, C. et al. (1984) Analysis of the ingredients of Angelica sinensis. Kexue Tongbao (Foreign Lang. Ed.) 29:560-562.

ANALYSIS

Product	Dong Quai, Chinese Angelica
Type	Standardized extract
Quality	traditional
Color	brownish powder
Taste	bitter sweet, warm and aromatic
Standardization	1% Ligustilide
pH	5.72
Ash	2.41%
Loss on drying:	2.52%
Heavy Metals	<20 ppm
Lead	1.2 ppm
Arsenic	<1 ppm
Microbiological Specifications	<1000 g
E. coli	<10 ppg.
S. aureus	< 50 ppg.
Salmonella	none
yeasts & moulds	< 10 ppg.
Particle size	100% pass through 30 mesh sieve
Pesticides	complies
Solvent residues	absent
Foreign matter	absent
Bulk density: loose	0.71
packed	0.79

ECHINACEA

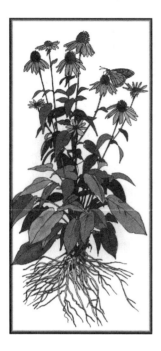

COMMON NAME
Echinacea, Black Sampson, Purple Coneflower, Rudbeckia, Missouri snakeroot

LATIN NAME
Echinacea purpurea,
E. angustifolia, E. pallida

ORIGIN
USA, cultivated in Eastern Europe

PART OF THE PLANT USED
root and rhizome

ACTIVE SUBSTANCES
polysaccharides (echinacin) echinacosides, caffeic acid glycoside, essential oil (humulene, caryophylene), polyacetylenes, isobutyl-alkylamines, resin, betain, insulin, sesquiterpene esters (Echinadiole, Epoxy-echinadiole, Echinaxanthole, Dihydro-xynardole).

STANDARDS
(1) Angustifolia
4% echinacosides (*E. angustifolia*) or 4% 4-Sesquiterpene-esters (*E. purpurea*)
(2) Angustifolia and Purpurea Combination

DESCRIPTION
Echinacea was the remedy of the Native American Indians from the Plains for wounds, infections, and insect and snake bites. The purple Coneflower is a member of the sunflower family. The three most common species are *Echinacea angustifolia*, *E. purpurea*, and *E. pallida*. In the United States, the roots of *E. angustifolia* have been used traditionally. Europe has performed more studies with fresh plant extracts of *E. purpurea*.

PHARMACOLOGY
Echinacea is rich in polysaccharides and phytosterols which have potent non-specific stimulatory actions on the immune system. Research has indicated that they stimulate the Alternative Complement pathway which helps activate general immune cells to scavenge for bacteria and cellular debris. The roots of *E. angustifolia* contain significant amounts of the glycoside echinacoside. Echinacoside has mild antibiotic activity. Other components in echinacea, such as the polysaccharide echinacin, also have antibiotic and antifungal activity. *E. purpurea* contains components, mainly echinacin, with cortisone-like activity and which help with wound healing by inhibiting inflammatory hyaluronidase enzyme. *E. purpurea* also contains the sesquiterpene esters which have immunostimulatory activity.

HISTORICAL USES

- Immune stimulator for colds and flus, sluggish immune systems
- Inflammation, analgesic, sedative, anti-spasmodic
- Relieve pain and swelling
- Edema, water retention
- Anti-viral
- Infections, sore throats, UTI, strep throat; eye and ear infections
- Wound healing and cleansing
- Anti-cancer
- Snake and insect bites, scratches
- Boils, abscesses, gangrene, ulcerations, sores
- Tonsillitis, inflamed gums, mucus problems
- Urticaria (external wash)
- Antibiotic
- Allergies
- Stimulation of adrenal cortex, increase cortisol release

ECHINACEA

DIRECTIONS FOR USE

250 mg. extract or 1 gm. root, increase during flu season up to 1000 mg. extract. For maintenance purposes, use periodically for a few weeks at a time.

BIO-ENHANCING AGENTS:

Goldenseal, ginseng, astragalus, licorice

TOXICITY, CAUTIONS & CONTRA-INDICATIONS

No observed toxicity. Side effects are rare. Persons with kidney disorders should restrict usage to 10 days of intake due to possible imbalance in excreted minerals.

PROCESSING

Cold water/ethanol extraction (repercolation). Evaporation at low temperature, low pressure.

SCIENTIFIC REFERENCES

• Foster, S. (1991) Echinacea, The Purple Coneflower. American Botanical Council, No. 301.
• Hobbs, C. (1989) The Echinacea handbook. Portland, OR: Eclectic Medical Publication.
• Mowrey, D. (1990) Guaranteed Potency Herbs. A Compilation of writings on the subject.
• Mowrey, D. (1986) The Scientific Validation of Herbal Medicine. Cormorant Books.
• Samochowiez, E. et al. (1979) Evaluation of the effect of Calendula officinalis and Echinacea angustifolia on Trichomonus vaginalis in vitro. Wiadmosci Parazytologiczne. 25(1):77.
• Tragni, E. et al. (1985) Evidence from two classic irritation tests for an anti-inflammatory action of a natural extract, Echinacin B. Food and Chem. Toxic. 23(1):317.
• Wacker, A. and Hilbig, A. (1978) Virus inhibition by Echinacea purpurea. Planta Medica 33:89.
• Wagner, H. and Proksch, A. (1981) An immunostimulating active principle from Echinacea purpurea. Angew. Phytother. 2(5):166.
• Weiner, M. (1990) Weiner's Herbal. Mill Valley: Quantum Books.

ANALYSIS

Product #1	Black Sampson, *Echinacea* toot
Type	Standardized extract
Quality	traditional
Color	brown fine powder
Standardization	4.27 % echinacosides
TLC ID	complies
pH (10% solution)	5.32 (5.0 -6.5)
Water (K. Fischer)	1.00
Total Ash	.62%
Heavy Metals	No more than 20 ppm
Microbiological Specifications	absent
Bacteria	<=1000.0 cfu/g
Fungi	<=100.0 cfu/g
Storage	Store sealed in a cool dry place
Product #2 Combination	Echinacea angustofolia and purpurea
Type	Standardized Extract
Quality	Traditional;
Color	Tan
Standardization	4% extract (echinacosides, cichoric acid, chlorogenic acid)
Solubility	Sparingly
Loss on drying	4.3%
Microbiological Specifications	absent
Aerobic Plate Count	<=10,000.0 cfu/g
E. coli	neg
Salmonella	neg
Yeast, Mold	<=100.0 cfu/g
Storage	Store sealed in a cool dry place

ACTIVE PROPERTIES

Echinacea has been used to boost the immune system, to help speed wound healing, to reduce inflammations, and to treat colds, flus and infections. Many of the active components of echinacea have antibacterial, antiviral, and antifungal properties. Echinacea has also been used externally to cleanse and heal wounds, eczema, burns, psoriasis, herpes, vaginitis, canker sores, abscesses, and other skin conditions. Recent research has indicated that echinacea has potent anti-tumor activity and helps stimulate the immune system to destroy cancer cells.

EPHEDRA

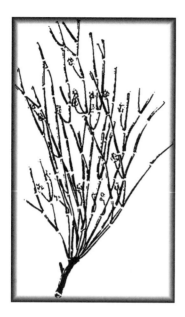

COMMON NAME
Ma Huang, Chinese Ephedra, Mormon tea, Squaw Tea
LATIN NAME
Ephedra sinica. E. girardiana, E. equisatina, E. dystachia
ORIGIN
China, India, Middle East
PART OF PLANT USED
Herb, Stems, Leaves (overground parts)
ACTIVE SUBSTANCES
Ephedrine, pseudo-ephedrine, norephedrine, methylephedrine, tannins, saponin, flavone, catechins, terpenol
STANDARD
5.5-6.5% Alkaloids (Ephedrine and pseudo-ephedrine)

DESCRIPTION
Ephedra or Ma Huang is a perennial herb belonging to the gymnosperms. The plant is made up of slender aerial green stems with small vestigial leaves. Ephedra has been used in Chinese medicine for thousands of years for bronchial spasms and as a stimulant for the sympathetic nervous system.

PHARMACOLOGY
Ephedra is a source of ephedrine, an alkaloid similar to adrenaline in its ability to excite the sympathetic nervous system. Ephedrine was used earlier in the century as a cure for asthma since it relaxes airways. But the isolated drug fell into disfavor when it was found to raise blood pressure. The whole plant however contains a mixture of alkaloids which counteract the activities of ephedrine, resulting in a safer and more balanced action. Ephedradines and pseudo-ephedrine lower blood pressure and reduce heart rate while still relaxing smooth muscle and opening the respiratory system.

ACTIVE PROPERTIES/
Ephedra has been used in China and Europe to treat asthma, hayfever, allergies, and arthritis, to break fevers, clear blocked sinuses, raise blood pressure, and increase alertness and perception. Ephedra is a stimulant of the sympathetic nervous system which controls the "Fight or Flight" response of the body.

PROCESSING
Ephedra stems are collected and dried. Autumn harvests contain the highest alkaloid content. The stems are concentrated in a similar manner to traditional methods with a water/ethanol extraction at low temperature, then evaporation at low temperature and pressure to create a natural extract standardized for total alkaloid content with all the other plant constituents included.

DIRECTIONS FOR USE
1 gm./day dried herb, corresponds to approx. 200 mg. of extract.

HISTORICAL USES

- Bronchodilator
- Circulatory system stimulant
- Appetite reducer
- Diuretic
- Anti-allergic
- Cough in feverish states
- Asthma bronchial, catarrh in upper respiratory tract
- Urticaria
- Enuresis
- Hypotension
- Nasal congestion
- Chills and "cold" fevers

EPHEDRA

TOXICITY, CAUTIONS & CONTRA-INDICATIONS

Contraindicated at high or medium elevated blood pressure. Should not be taken together with other CNS stimulants or circulatory agents (digitoxin, beta-blockers, etc.). A single high dose could result in irregular heart beats.

SCIENTIFIC REFERENCES

• Morton, J. (1977) Major medicinal plants. Springfield, Ill: Charles C. Thomas.
• Duke, J. (1988) CRC Handbook of Medicinal herbs. Boca Raton, Florida: CRC Press.

ANALYSIS

Product	Ephedra, Ma Huang
Type	standardized extract
Standard	5.5-6.5% alkaloids
Method	DAB 9 German Pharmacopoiea method, HPLC
Color	fine mid-brown powder
Characteristic	good flow
Flavor	bitter and aromatic
pH	5.2-5.5
Ash	no more than 7 %
Loss on drying (vacuum at 100-105°C)	no more than 7 %
Heavy Metals	no more than 25 ppm
Storage	Seal in a cool dry, dark place

FEVERFEW

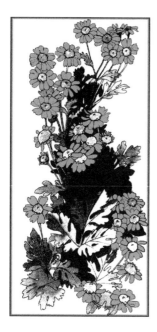

COMMON NAME
Feverfew
LATIN NAME
Tanacetum parthenium
ORIGIN
German, Holland, UK, Israel
PART OF PLANT USED
Leaves
ACTIVE SUBSTANCES
Sesquiterpene lactones (including parthenolide, chrysanthemonin, chrysartemin A and B, and santamarin), tannins, beta-farnesene, camphor.
STAN DARD
0.1- 0.5% parthenolide

DESCRIPTION
Feverfew was known to the ancient Egyptians and Greeks as a valuable herbal remedy, used as an anti-inflammatory agent, to treat headaches, and as an emmenagogue (promoting menstrual flow). Feverfew is a member of the daisy family, similar to the tansy and chrysanthemum. The herb has become popular with the recent clinical trials showing its effectiveness as a remedy for migraine headaches.

PHARMACOLOGY
Feverfew contains the bitter-tasting sesquiterpene lactones of which parthenolide is the most pharmacologically active. Research studies determined that parthenolide, michefuscalide, and chrysanthenyl acetate inhibited the production of prostaglandins. This inhibition of prostaglandins results in reduction in inflammation, decreased secretion of histamine, decreased activation of inflammatory cells and a reduction of fever, from whence the name of the herb. This reduction of prostaglandins and histamines is thought to be part of the reason for the efficacy of feverfew in treating migraines by reducing spasms of blood vessels.

ACTIVE PROPERTIES
With its anti-inflammatory activities, Feverfew has also been useful against swellings and arthritis; for relaxing the smooth muscles in the uterus, promoting menstrual flow; and for inhibiting platelet aggregation and excessive blood clotting. As a bitter herb, feverfew has also been useful in stimulating digestion and improving the functioning of the liver.

PROCESSING
Leaves are harvested and extracted. The extract is concentrated to arrive at the guaranteed potency.

DIRECTIONS FOR USE
One capsule of extract containing 500 mg. parthenolide. For migraines, needs to be taken for an entire month before effects are noticed.

HISTORICAL USES

- Inflammations, hot swellings
- Migraines, tension headaches
- Nausea, vomiting
- Vertigo
- Arthritis
- Depression
- Acute fever
- Asthma
- Menstrual difficulties
- As an emmenagogue
- As a liver tonic
- To aid digestion
- To promote restful sleep

FEVERFEW

BIO-ENHANCING AGENTS
skullcap, rosemary leaf

**TOXICITY, CAUTIONS &
CONTRA-INDICATIONS**
No toxicity seen in clinical trials.

SCIENTIFIC REFERENCES

• Weiner, M. (1990) Weiner's Herbal.
Mill Valley, CA:Quantum Books.
• Grieve, M. (1978) A Modern Herbal.
Middlesex, UK: Penguin Books.
• Heptinstall, S. (1988) Feverfew-- An
ancient remedy for modern times? J. Royal
Soc. Med. 81:373-374.
• Bohlmann, F. and Zdero, C. (1982)
Sesquiterpene lactones and other constitu-
ents from Tanacetum parthenum. Phyto-
chemistry 21:2543.
• Makheja, A. and Bailey, J. (1981) The
active principle of Feverfew. Lancet
2:1054.
• Johnson, E.S. et al. (1985) Efficacy of
Feverfew as prophylactic treatment of
migraine. Brit. Med. J. 291:569.
• Murphy, J.J et al. (1988) Randomised
double-blind trial of Feverfew in migraine
prevention. The Lancet 2:189.

ANALYSIS

Analysis	Result
Total Sesquiterpene Lactones (calculated as Parthenolide)	0.13%
Total Sesquiterpene Lactones (calculated in dry extract)	0.4%
Ratio plant to extract	3
pH	5.3
Ash	6.2%
Heavy metals	conforms
Microbiology	conforms

CHINESE GARLIC

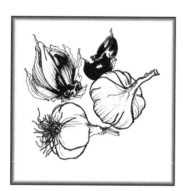

COMMON NAME
Garlic
LATIN NAME
Allium sativum
ORIGIN:
China (Xianjiang province)
PART OF PLANT USED
Cloves
ACTIVE SUBSTANCES
Alliin, Allinase, Allicin, vitamins A, B, C
STANDARD
12 mg/g Alliin, 90% Allinase activity, 4000 mcg Total Allicin Potential (TAP)

DESCRIPTION

Garlic is a perennial plant with white, starry flowers and bulb clusters of individual cloves. The plant has been used for both culinary and medical reasons. The plant has been used to protect against infections, to lower blood cholesterol and fat levels, and to help with digestion. Modern research has confirmed these effects. The Chinese have valued garlic for thousands of years for its extraordinary healing properties and have recently discovered a unique and meticulous way to process the garlic cloves in order to stabilize the active ingredients and to maximize the Total Allicin Potential (TAP) that reaches the consumer.

PHARMACOLOGY

The principle active agent in garlic is alliin. When garlic cloves are cut or bruised, the alliin is converted to the pungent-smelling allicin by the action of the enzyme allinase. Extreme care must be taken during processing of the cloves to maximize the TAP of garlic. Any bruising of the cloves or harsh treatment would result in conversion of the alliin to allicin and loss of the active ingredients. Alliin and Allicin are sulphur-containing components. The sulphur compounds have antibiotic and antifungal effects. They help stop the liver from making too much cholesterol and reduce clotting tendencies.

DIRECTIONS FOR USE

400 mg/day standardized extract equivalent to 1200 mg of fresh garlic

BIO-ENHANCING AGENTS

Vitamin C, chlorophyll, parsley

TOXICITY, CAUTIONS & CONTRA-INDICATIONS

No toxicity reported.

PROCESSING

Chinese Garlic is meticulously dried at ultra-low temperature to protect the TAP and enzyme activity. The powder is compressed into tablets and coated with an enteric coating and a clear protein coating to lock in freshness and to eliminate odor.

HISTORICAL USE

- To protect and fight against infections, colds, flus
- Antibiotic, antifungal, antiviral, anti-candida, anti-worms, antiparasitic, antiprotozoan
- Expectorant, reduce phlegm, bronchitis, asthma, pneumonia
- Protect wounds from infection, treat abscesses, cuts
- Protect the circulation, lower cholesterol and fat levels
- Thin the blood, thrombosis, reduce blood clotting
- Lower blood sugar levels
- Antitoxin (carcinogens, heavy metals, drugs, poisons)
- Stimulate and protect the liver
- Anti-cancer
- Digestive tonic, gastritis, dysentery
- To ward off vampires and protect from black magic

CHINESE GARLIC

SCIENTIFIC REFERENCES
• Bordia, A. (1981) Effect of garlic on blood lipids in patients with coronary heart disease. Amer. J. Clin. Nutr. 34(10):2100.
• Bordia, A. and Bansal, H. C. (1973) Essential oil of garlic in prevention of atherosclerosis. Lancet ii:1491.
• McCaleb, R. (1992) Garlic fantastic health aid. Better Nutrition for Today's Living. Feb 92:36.
• Mowrey, D. (1986) The Scientific Validation of Herbal Medicine. Cormorant Books.
• Nishimo, H. et al. (1989) Antitumor-Promoting activity of garlic extracts. Oncology 46(4):277.
• Weiner, M. (1990) Weiner's Herbal. Mill Valley: Quantum Books.

ANALYSIS

Description	
Moisture	4.9%
Color	White
Shape/size	7/16" round
Thickness	0.265" - 0.275"
Hardness	8 -10 kg
Average tablet wt.	700 mg
Variation	+ - 5%
Assay results	
Garlic	400 mg
Coating	enteric coated
Total Allicin Potential	11.6 mg/g

GINGER

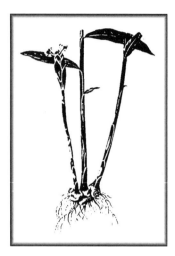

COMMON NAME
Ginger
LATIN NAME
Zingiber officinale
ORIGIN
Israel, China, India, Nigeria
PART OF PLANT USED
Rhizomes
ACTIVE SUBSTANCES
Phenylalkylketones (Gingerols, Shogaols, Zingerone); volatile oil (zingiberone, bisabolene, camphene, geranial, linalool, borneol)
STANDARD
5% of total pungent compounds including the phenylalkylketones (particularly the two main, 3-methoxy-4 hydroxy aromatic compounds 6-gingerol and 6-shogaol) or 4% volatile oils

DESCRIPTION
Ginger is one of the most widely used roots both for culinary purposes and for medicinal ones. Recent medical studies have confirmed the ancient uses of Ginger as a carminative, cholalogue, antitussive, diaphoretic, and to help the absorption of other remedies throughout the body.

PHARMACOLOGY
The main components of Ginger are the aromatic essential oil, antioxidants, and the pungent oleoresin. The pungent compounds have been identified as the phenylalkylketones, known as gingerols, shogaols, and zingerone.

ACTIVE PROPERTIES
Most of the medicinal effects of ginger appear to be due to the pungent components which are standardized. Recent research published in Lancet and other prestigious journals have confirmed the traditional uses for ginger. Ginger was found more effective than drugs at treating motion sickness and nausea. Ginger is able to calm the stomach, promote bile flow, and improve the appetite. Ginger is also known for its warming expectorant action on the upper respiratory tract, suppressing coughs, and encouraging the release of mucus and phlegm. With its diaphoretic action, promoting sweating, and increasing circulation, it is additionally useful for colds and low grade fevers. Ginger tea has long been a standard remedy for sore throats, colds and flus. Recent studies have found that Ginger lowers blood cholesterol and reduces blood clotting. The pungent compound, gingerol has been found to have a structure similar to the well-known anticoagulant, aspirin, which may explain the similar effect that the two compounds have on prostaglandins. Ginger is also a very effective antibiotic agent and strong anti-oxidant.

HISTORICAL USES

- Nausea, vomiting, motion sickness, vertigo, morning sickness
- Loss of appetite
- Stomach ache, dyspepsia, flatulence, indigestion
- To promote bile flow
- Colds, coughs, influenza, fevers
- High cholesterol
- As an antioxidant
- To thin the blood, as an anti-coagulant

GINGER

PROCESSING

Alcohol/water extraction process. A specially developed micro-encapsulation procedure preserves the volatile active ingredients within a free flowing powder. The extract is concentrated about 3 times compared to dry ginger and 30 times compared to fresh ginger. The concentration of gingerols is determined by nuclear magnetic resonance techniques (NMR).

DIRECTIONS FOR USE

500 mg./day extract or 1.5 gm./day dry ginger

TOXICITY, CAUTIONS & CONTRA-INDICATIONS

No toxicity known.

SCIENTIFIC REFERENCES

• Mowrey, D. (1986) The Scientific Validation of Herbal Medicine. Cormorant Books.
• Govindarajan, V.S. (1982) Ginger - Chemistry, Technology, and Quality Evaluation. CRC Critical Rev. in Food Science and Nutrition. 17(3).
• Lee, Y.B. et al. (1986) Antioxidant property in Ginger rhizomes and its application to meat products. J. of Food Sci. 51:20-23.
• Mowrey, D. and Clayson, D.E. (1982) Motion sickness, Ginger and psychophysics. Lancet Mar. 20, i:655-657.
• Gujral, S. et al. (1978) Effect of ginger (Zingiber officinale roscoe) oleoresin on serum and hepatic cholesterol levels in cholesterol fed rats. Nutrition Reports Intern. 17(2), 183-189.
• Yamahara, J. et al. (1985) Cholagogic effects of Ginger and its active constituents. J. Ethnopharm. 113:217-225.
• Shoji, N. et al. (1982) Cardiotonic principles of Ginger (Zingiber officinale Roscoe). J. Pharm. Sci. 71:1174-1175.

ANALYSIS

Product	Zingiber officinale, Roscoe; Ginger Root
Type	Standardized extract
Standardization	6% gingerols, shogaols, and zingerone
Appearance	free flowing tan colored powder
Loss on drying	3.28%
Taste	warm, pungent, aromatic, characteristic
Ash	1.67%
pH	4.72
Mesh size	conforms
Heavy Metals	not more than 15 ppm
Pesticides	<specifications
Microbiology:Total count	<1,000 cfu/g
E. coli	<10
Coliform	<30
S. Aureus	<10
Salmonella	neg
Yeasts and Molds	<20
Storage	

GINKGO BILOBA

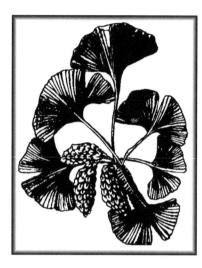

COMMON NAME
Ginkgo biloba,
Maidenhair Tree
LATIN NAME
Ginkgo biloba
ORIGIN
China, Japan, Worldwide
PART OF PLANT USED
Leaves
ACTIVE SUBSTANCES
ginkgoflavoglycosides
(kaempferol, quercetin,
isorhamnetin, prontho-
cyanidins), terpenes
(Ginkgolides, bilobalides)
STANDARD
24% ginkgo flavoglycosides

DESCRIPTION
Ginkgo biloba is one of the world's oldest living tree species, believed to have survived for 200 million years. Individual trees have lived 1000 years. Ginkgo trees are tall hardy trees, highly resistant to pollutants and pests with distinctive fan-shaped leaves. Ginkgo is considered a sacred tree by the Chinese and has been used in Oriental Medicine since ancient times for respiratory ailments and for brain function. Hundreds of studies have been performed with Ginkgo biloba extracts confirming many of the ancient uses as well as finding new applications.

PHARMACOLOGY
The main active compounds in Ginkgo leaves are the flavoglycosides: kaempferol, quercetin, isorhamnetin, and proanthocyanidins. These compounds have anti-oxidant and free radical properties. Also important are the terpenes: ginkgolides and bilobalides.

HISTORICAL USE

One way these agents decrease inflammation is by inhibiting Platelet Activating Factor (PAF) and reducing the stickiness of platelets which can result in decreased circulatory flow. PAF has been implicated in a wide variety of diseases including asthma, heart arrhythmias, myocardial infarction, and atherosclerosis.

ACTIVE PROPERTIES
Numerous studies have detailed the efficacy of Ginkgo biloba extract (GBE) for a wide variety of conditions. GBE has been reported to increase circulation to the brain and thus help with cases of dementia, Alzheimer's disease, memory loss, concentration problems, vertigo, tinnitus, and dizziness. Peripheral vascular diseases such as Raynaud's syndrome, intermittent claudication, numbness, tingling have been helped by GBE. Studies have also reported that GBE was helpful in cases of head injuries, macular degeneration, asthma, and impotence.

- Cerebral vascular insufficiency, vertigo, headaches, tinnitus
- Mental performance, brain function, concentration problems
- Senility, memory loss, dementia, Alzheimer's, dizziness
- Peripheral arterial insufficiency
- Peripheral vascular diseases, Raynaud's syndrome, numbness, tingling
- Ischemia
- Edema
- Hypoxia
- Impotence and erectile dysfunction
- Hemorrhoids
- Inflammation
- Migraine
- Inflammation
- Allergies
- Asthma

GINKGO BILOBA

BIO-ENHANCING AGENTS
Bilberry, Butcher's Broom, Centella, Milk Thistle, Vitamin B complex, magnesium, choline, inositol

TOXICITY, CAUTIONS & CONTRA-INDICATIONS
No reported toxicity. Rare cases of gastric upset or headaches.

PROCESSING
Green leaves are harvested in the fall and air dried, then extracted in water/acetone mixture, filtered and concentrated.

DIRECTIONS FOR USE
120 mg daily

SCIENTIFIC REFERENCES

• Bauer, U. (1984) 6 Month double-blind randomized clinical trial of Ginkgo biloba extract versus placebo in two parallel groups of patients suffering from peripheral arterial insufficiency. Arzneim.-Forsch./Drug Res. 34:716.
• Brown, D. (1992) Ginkgo Biloba-Old and New: Part I. Let's Live 60(4):46.
Chung, K. F. et al. (1987) Effect of a ginkgolide mixture (BN 52063) in antagonizing skin and platelet responses to platelet activating factor in man. Lancet, Jan 31.
• Hindmarch, I. (1986) Activite de l'extrait de Ginkgo biloba sur la memoire a court terme/ Activity of Ginkgo Biloba extract on short term memory. Presse Medicale. 15:1592.
• Kleijnen, J. and Knipschild, P. (1992) Ginkgo biloba. Lancet 340(7):1136.
• Mowrey, D. (1988) Guaranteed Potency Herbs. Next Generation Herbal Medicine. Lehi, UT:Cormorant Books.
• Sikora, R. et al. (1989) Ginkgo biloba extract in the therapy of erectile dysfunction. J. Urol. 141:188A.
• Vorberg, G. (1985) GBE: long term study concerning the major symptoms of age-related cerebral disorders. Clin. Trials. J. 22:149.
• Weiner, M. (1990) Weiner's Herbal. Mill Valley: Quantum Books.

ANALYSIS

Product:	Ginkgo Biloba Dry Extract
Type	Standardized extract
Standardization	Ginkgoflavonglycosides 24.5%
Total Terpene Lactones	6.5%
Ginkgolide A	1.8%
Ginkgolide B	0.8%
Ginkgolide C	0.7%
Bilobalide	3.0%
Loss on drying:	2.5%
Ash	0.71%
Heavy Metals	<20 ppm
Microbiological Specifications (Pharm. Acta. Helv. 51(3):33-40. 1976)	
Gram negatives	absent
Escherichia coli	absent
Staphylococcus aureus	absent
Pseudomonas aeruginosa	absent
Salmonella sp.	absent

AMERICAN GINSENG

(*Panax quinquefolium*)

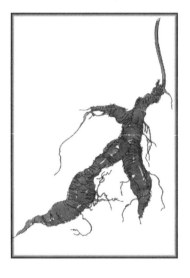

COMMON NAME
Ginseng, American ginseng
LATIN NAME
Panax quinquefolium
ORIGIN
Canada, eastern US, Wisconsin, China
PART OF PLANT USED
Root
ACTIVE SUBSTANCES
Glycosides (Ginsenosides), saponins, phytosterol
STANDARD
5-15% ginsenosides, mainly Rb1

DESCRIPTION

Panax quinquefolium is a deciduous perennial shrub whose fleshy root requires 4 years of cultivation to reach maturity. Traditionally the wild root was consumed by American Indians as a general tonic, as a natural restorative for weak and wounded, and to help the mind. American ginseng is now used as a natural preventive and restorative remedy and valued for its adaptogenic properties. American ginseng (*Panax quinquefolium*) is more sedative and relaxing and increases "yin" energy while Korean ginseng is more stimulating and increases the "yang" energy. American ginseng is suitable for females and young people as well as males and older people.

PHARMACOLOGY

The main active ingredients of ginseng are the more than 20 saponin triterpenoid glycosides called ginsenosides whose names relate to their chromatographic position (Ra, Rb, etc.). American ginseng is rich in the Rb1 group of ginsenosides which have more sedative and metabolic effects on the central nervous system, compared to the Rg1 group of ginsenosides which are more arousing and stimulating. Rb1 Ginsenosides have CNS-depressing activity, have weak anti-inflammatory action, and increase digestive tract peristalsis. Laboratory animals given Rb1 ginsenosides have improved stamina and increased learning abilities. Other studies have shown that Rb1 ginsenosides also have anti-fatigue, anti-convulsant, antipyretic, antipsychotic, analgesic, and ulcer protective effects.

ACTIVE PROPERTIES

American ginseng has been used for stress and fatigue characterized by insomnia, poor appetite, nervousness, and restlessness. The root has been used for conditions

HISTORICAL USES

- CNS depressant, anticon-vulsant, analgesic, tranquilizing
- Sedative, relaxant
- Anti-fatigue (insomnia, nervousness, poor appetite)
- Restorative for active or nervous, agitated disposition
- Increase vitality in conditions of weakness, prolonged stress, poor immunity, or chronic disease
- Hypotensive
- Anti-stress
- Anti-psychotic
- Anti-inflammatory and anti-pyretic
- Increase gastro-intestinal motility
- Increase synthesis of cholesterol in liver
- Immune system stimulant
- Regulate adrenal gland, inhibit exhaustion of gland
- Regulate blood sugar and lipid levels
- Anti-tumor

AMERICAN GINSENG

(Panax quinquefolium)

of weakness, convalescence, low resistance, poor immunity or debility due to chronic disease. Scientific support is now emerging for its use in the regulation of various metabolic disturbances including blood sugar and lipid levels.

DIRECTIONS FOR USE
500-600 mg. extract)/day
1-2 gm/day dried root

TOXICITY, CAUTIONS & CONTRA-INDICATIONS
No reported toxicity.

PROCESSING
4 year old roots are harvested and dried.

SCIENTIFIC REFERENCES
• Baldwin, CS et al. (1986) What pharmacists should know about Ginseng. Pharm. J. Nov 8th:582.
• Brekhman, I.I. and Dardymov, I.V. (1969) New substances of plant origin which increase nonspecific resistance. Ann Rev Pharm. 9:419.
• Hia, et al. (1979) Stimulation of pituitary adrenocortical system by ginseng saponins. Endocrinol. Japonica. 26(6):661.
• Mowrey, D. (1990) Guaranteed Potency Herbs. A Compilation of writings on the subject.
• Oshima, Y et al. (1987) J. Nat. Prod. 50:188.
• Weiner, M. (1990) Weiner's Herbal. Mill Valley: Quantum Books.

ANALYSIS

Type	Standardized extract
Standardization	
15.11 (>=14.0)	Ginsenoside Rg1- 1.57%
	Ginsenoside Rb1 - 3.05%
	ratio Rg1/Rb1 51-47%
Character	brown-yellow amorphous powder
Loss on drying:	3.85 (<=7.0)
pH	5.35 (4.0 - 6.0)
Ash	6.29 (<=9.0)
Heavy Metals	<50.0 (<=50.0) ppm
Total residual organic solvents	0.1 (<=2.0)
Total Aerobic Microbial count	<1000.0 (<=1000.0) cfu/g
fungi	<100.0 (<=100.0) cfu/g
staph aureus, salmonella	absent
E. coli	absent

KOREAN GINSENG

(*Panax ginseng*)

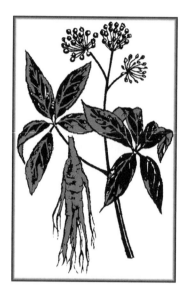

COMMON NAME
Ginseng, Asian ginseng,
Korean ginseng, Asiatic ginger, Chinese ginseng,
Wonder-of-the-world

LATIN NAME
Panax ginseng

ORIGIN
Asian mountain forests,
Korea

PART OF PLANT USED
Root

ACTIVE SUBSTANCE
Glycosides (Ginsenosides),
saponins, phytosterol

STANDARD
15% ginsenosides,
mainly Rg1

DESCRIPTION

Panax ginseng is a deciduous perennial shrub whose fleshy root requires 4-6 years of cultivation to reach maturity. Traditionally the wild root was consumed to vitalize, strengthen, and rejuvenate the entire body. Widely cultivated, ginseng is now used as a natural preventive, restorative remedy and valued for its adaptogenic properties. Korean ginseng is more stimulating and increases the "yang" energy while American ginseng (*Panax quinquefolium*) increases the "yin" energy. Korean ginseng is most suitable for males and older people.

PHARMACOLOGY

The main active ingredients of ginseng are the more than 20 saponin triterpenoid glycosides called ginsenosides whose names relate to their chromatographic position (Ra, Rb, etc.). Rb1 group of ginsenosides have more sedative and metabolic effects on the central nervous system, while the Rg1 group of ginsenosides are more arousing and stimulating at low doses. Rb1 Ginsenosides have CNS-depressing activity, have weak anti-inflammatory action, and increase digestive tract peristalsis. Other studies have shown that Rb1 ginsenosides also are anti-convulsant, antipyretic, anti-psychotic, analgesic, and ulcer protective. These activities contrast with those of Rg1 ginsenosides which have weak CNS-stimulating activity, protect against fatigue, and cause an increase in motor activity. *Panax ginseng* (Korean) contains higher amounts of the more stimulating Rg1 ginsenosides compared to American ginseng (*Panax quinquefolium*) which has a higher amount of the more sedative Rb1 ginsenosides. Both Rg1 and Rb1 ginsenosides act on the adrenal and pituitary glands and help them respond to stress more rapidly.

HISTORICAL USES

- Adaptogen, general tonic
- Anti-stress
- Anti-fatigue, restore vigor
- Restorative
- Increase resistance to infections
- Slight CNS stimulant
- Increase mental and physical work capacity
- Increase concentration and mental activity
- Enhance mental acuity and intellectual performance
- Improve physical performance
- Immunoregulator, mainly immunostimulant
- Promote appetite
- Anti-oxidant
- Increase reaction times
- Lower blood cholesterol
- Radioprotective
- Regulates adrenal glands, helps prevent exhaustion

KOREAN GINSENG

(Panax ginseng)

ACTIVE PROPERTIES
Korean Ginseng is used for conditions of tiredness, weakness, debility, convalescence, low resistance, aging, stress, poor metabolism, and lack of concentration. Ginseng extracts have been shown to have antioxidant activity and to protect against radiation damage. European clinical trials have found an increase in reaction times, alertness, concentration, and visual and motor coordination.

DIRECTIONS FOR USE
500-600 mg./day of extract;
1-2 gm./day dried root

BIO-ENHANCING AGENTS
Licorice

TOXICITY, CAUTIONS & CONTRA-INDICATIONS
No reported adverse effects. May cause a slight insomnia if taken at bedtime. A report by Siegal, entitled The Ginseng Abuse Syndrome, has been shown to have no merit.

PROCESSING
Six-year roots are harvested and extracted, then standardized at 23-27% ginsenosides and ratio between Rb1 content and Rg1 content not exceeding 2.

SCIENTIFIC REFERENCES
• Baldwin, CS et al. (1986) What pharmacists should know about Ginseng. Pharm. J. Nov 8th:582.
• Brekhman, I.I. and Dardymov, I.V. (1969) New substances of plant origin which increase nonspecific resistance. Ann Rev Pharm. 9:419.
• Hia, et al. (1979) Stimulation of pituitary adrenocortical system by ginseng saponins. Endocrinol. Japonica. 26(6):661.
• Mowrey, D. (1990) Guaranteed Potency Herbs. A Compilation of writings on the subject.
• Shibata, S. et al. (1985) Chemistry and pharmacology of Panax. In: Economic and Medicinal Plant Research, Vol. 1.
• Weiner, M. (1990) Weiner's Herbal. Mill Valley: Quantum Books.

ANALYSIS

Product:	
Type	Standardized extract
Standardization	15% ginsenosides
Character	Cream
Taste	bitter and slightly sweet with an aromatic undertone
Loss on drying:	3.12%
pH	6.13
Ash	6.93%
Pesticide residues	conforms/none detected
Heavy Metals	no more than 5 ppm
Microbiological Specifications: Total Viable Count	<10 cfu/g
Escherichia coli	<10
Coliform	<10
Staphylococcus aureus	<10
Salmonella sp.	neg
Yeasts and Molds	<10

SIBERIAN GINSENG

(*Eleutherococcus senticosus*)

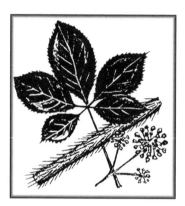

COMMON NAME
Siberian Ginseng, Ciwujia, Devil's Shrub, Touch-Me-Not, Ussurian thorny pepperbush

LATIN NAME
Eleutherococcus senticosus (or *Acanthopanax senticosus*)

ORIGIN
China, Russia (Eastern Siberia), Manchuria, Korea

PART OF PLANT USED
Rhizome (underground creeping stem) and Roots

ACTIVE SUBSTANCES
Glycosides (Eleutherosides), resins, anthocyanin, pectin

STANDARD
0.3 % Eleutheroside B and 0.5 % Eleutheroside E
Total 0.8% Eleutherosides

DESCRIPTION
Siberian Ginseng is a tall wild deciduous shrub with many stalks and a woody root (not the typical fleshy rootstocks of the other ginsengs). The root has been used for 2000 years in China as general preventative medicine and tonic. During this century, Siberian Ginseng has been extensively studied by Russian scientists. Numerous clinical trials have established that *E. senticosus* acts as an adaptogen and helps human beings handle stressful conditions and excel in athletic and mental endeavors.

PHARMACOLOGY
The eleutherosides have been shown to be responsible for the adaptogenic properties of the plant. The eleutherosides are a range of glycosides with aromatic alcohol aglycones. (Ginsenosides have triterpenoid aglycones) The glycosides appear to act on the adrenal glands, helping to prevent adrenal hypertrophy and excess corticosteroid production in response to stress. The eleutherosides additionally help reduce the exhaustion phase of the stress response and return the adrenals to normal function faster.

ACTIVE PROPERTIES
Siberian Ginseng is used by deep sea divers, long-distance drivers, mountain rescue workers, factory workers, athletes, submariners, and cosmonauts. After nearly a thousand studies, Siberian Ginseng has been shown to increase energy and stamina and to help the body resist viral infections, environmental toxins, radiation, and chemotherapy. In Chinese Medicine, *E. senticosus* has been used to prevent bronchial and other respiratory infections as well as viral infections. The Chinese used the root also to provide energy and vitality, to increase resistance, and to treat rheumatic diseases and heart ailments. Siberian Ginseng has been used in cardiovascular and neurovascular conditions to help restore memory, concentration, and cognitive abilities which may be impaired from poor

HISTORICAL USES

- Adaptogen
- Stress
- Fatigue, restore vigor
- Neurasthenia, debility, depression, nervous breakdown
- Allergies, hay fever
- Resistance to infections
- Normalize hypo- and hyperglycemia
- Increase mental and physical work capacity.
- Increase concentration, improve performance
- Reduce convalescence time
- Protect against environmental toxins and pollution
- Immunoregulator, mainly immunostimulant
- Promote appetite
- Increase fertility, for sterility

SIBERIAN GINSENG

(Eleutherococcus senticosus)

blood supply to the brain. Additionally Siberian Ginseng is a popular herbal remedy for debility, depression, fatigue, and nervous breakdowns.

DIRECTIONS FOR USE
500-600 mg. extract equiv to 2-5 gm./day dried plant

BIO-ENHANCING AGENTS
Ginkgo biloba

TOXICITY, CAUTIONS & CONTRA-INDICATIONS
No toxicity or side effects reported. Should not be taken with a high fever (above 39°C) or at a very high blood pressure (WHO stage 2).

PROCESSING
Two step repercolation at low temperature, made with different ethanol/water ratios and with pH stabilization to prevent hydrolysis of the eleutherosides. Evaporation at low temperature and low pressure.

SCIENTIFIC REFERENCES

• Brekhman, II. and Dardymov, IV. (1969) New substances of plant origin which increase nonspecific resistance. Ann Rev Pharm. 9:419.
• Farnsworth, NR. et al. (1985) Siberian Ginseng (Eleutherococcus senticosus): Current Status as an adaptogen. In H. Wagner, et al. (eds) Economic and Medicinal Plant Research. Vol. 1. Fl:Academic Press pp. 155-215.
• Foster, S. (1991) Siberian Ginseng (Eleutherococcus senticosus) American Botanical Council No. 302.
• Mowrey, D. (1990) Guaranteed Potency Herbs. A Compilation of writings on the subject.
• Mowrey, D. (1986) The Scientific Validation of Herbal Medicine. Cormorant Books.
• Weiner, M. (1990) Weiner's Herbal. Mill Valley: Quantum Books.

ANALYSIS

Product	Siberian Ginseng
Type	Standardized extract
Standardization	.46% Eleutheroside B, .63% Eleutheroside E
Character	light brown powder
Loss on drying	4.0%
pH	5.25
Ash	2.25%
Mesh size	conforms
Heavy Metals	conforms
Pestiside residues	conforms
Microbiological Specifications	
Escherichia coli	<10
Coliform	<30
Staphylococcus aureus	<10
Salmonella sp.	neg
Yeasts and Molds	<10

GOLDENSEAL

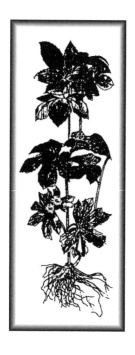

COMMON NAME
Goldenseal, yellow root, eye root, Indian turmeric, jaundice root
LATIN NAME
Hydrastis canadensis
ORIGIN
Northern America
PART OF PLANT USED
Rhizome (root-stock)
ACTIVE SUBSTANCES
alkaloids (Hydrastine, Berberine, Canadine, Berber-astine)
STANDARD
10% alkaloids (5% Hydrastine)

DESCRIPTION
Goldenseal root has been used by Native American healers for a wide range of ailments. The Indians used goldenseal for local inflammations and infections. The plant was also utilized to improve digestion as a bitter tonic and to treat ulcers. An infusion of the root was used as a soothing rinse for eye and skin infections.

PHARMACOLOGY
The active ingredients of goldenseal include a group of alkaloids, hydrastine and berberine. These alkaloids are strongly astringent and help reduce inflammation of mucous membranes. These alkaloids also have antiseptic properties. Hydrastine has been reported to lower blood pressure and stimulate peristalsis. Hydrastine is also anti-tussive. Berberine induces the secretion of bile and helps stop bleeding. A great deal of research has shown that berberine has anti-bacterial, anti-fungal and anti-parasitic activity. Goldenseal stimulates involuntary muscles through an oxytocic effect in the intestinal tract and uterus. The plant has been used during childbirth when the labor is protracted.

ACTIVE PROPERTIES
Goldenseal root has been recommended for a variety of inflamed mucous membranes, including stomach, intestinal, vaginal, and rectal. It has been reported that the plant relieves pains and helps heal wounds and stop bleeding. In addition the antibacterial action helps reduce or prevent infection of open sores. The Cherokee and Iroquois used the plant for diarrhea, dyspepsia, liver problems, flatulence, pneumonia, cancer, and rattlesnake bites. Modern uses have included as a laxative, for hemorrhoids, mouth sores, diuretic, eye infections, acne, sore throats, to ward off infections, and as an antiseptic.

HISTORICAL USES

- Inflammation of digestive system and mucous membranes
- Peptic ulcers, gastritis, flatulence, diarrhea, dyspepsia
- For liver and gall bladder problems
- Douche for Candida and thrush
- Skin infections, impetigo, ringworm, eczema
- To lower blood pressure
- As a sedative
- Anti-bacterial
- Anti-viral
- Vaginitis, gonorrhea, ureth-ritis and rectal inflammations
- Rhinitis
- Catarrhal conditions
- Eye inflammations
- Disturbances of endocrine and uterine function, for excessive menstruation and hemorrhaging

GOLDENSEAL

PROCESSING

Ethanol/water extraction at low temperature, pH adjusted to give maximum yield. Evaporation at low temperature and pressure.

DIRECTIONS FOR USE

250 mg. extract. Do not use for extended periods of time (greater than a week at a time).

BIO-ENHANCING AGENTS

Echinacea, garlic

TOXICITY, CAUTIONS & CONTRA-INDICATIONS

At doses of 2-3 gr. goldenseal can lower heart beat and at higher doses it can be paralyzing to the Central Nervous System (CNS). Do not use during pregnancy since Berberine stimulates the uterus. May induce abortion at high doses.

SCIENTIFIC REFERENCES

• Datta, D. et al. (1971) Thin layer chromatography and UV spectrophotometry of alcoholic extracts of Hydrastis canadensis. Planta Medica 19(3):258.
• Foster, S. (1991) Goldenseal. American Botanical Council, Botanical Series No. 309.
• Gupta, S. (1975) Use of berberine in the treatment of giardiasis. Amer. J. Dis. Childhood. 129:866.
• Ikram, M. (1975) A review of the chemical and pharmacological aspects of genus berberis. Planta Medica 28:353.
• Mowrey, D. (1990) Guaranteed Potency Herbs. A Compilation of writings on the subject.
• Mowrey, D. (1986) The Scientific Validation of Herbal Medicine. Cormorant Books.
• Sharda, D. (1970) Berberine in the treatment of diarrhea of infancy and childhood. J. Ind. Med. Assoc. 54(1):22.
• Weiner, M. (1990) Weiner's Herbal. Mill Valley: Quantum Books.

ANALYSIS

Determination Gravimetric Contents of total alkaloids calculated (hydrastine and berberine)	not < 10%
Color	green
TLC ID	complies
Total Aerobic Microbial count	<10,000.0 cfu/g
fungi	<100.0 cfu/g
staph areus, salmonella	absent
E. coli	absent
Coliform	absent
Yeasts and Molds	<100/g

GOTU KOLA
(CENTELLA ASIATICA)

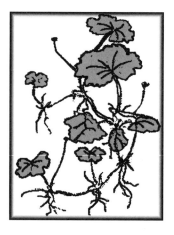

DESCRIPTION

Centella is actually a specific variety of gotu kola, but since no other varieties possess such high amounts of asiaticosides and other tri-terpenes, the term "centella" is reserved for just this variety; "gotu kola" is used for all other varieties. Centella is found only in Madagascar while the other varieties of gotu kola are found in India and neighboring countries. Centella does not contain caffeine or any derivatives.

PHARMACOLOGY

Asiaticosides stimulate the reticuloendothelial system where new blood cells are formed and old ones destroyed, fatty materials are stored, iron is metabolized, and immune responses and inflammation occur or begin. The primary mode of action of Centella appears to be on the various phases of connective tissue development, which are part of the healing process. Centella also increases keratinization, the process of building more skin in areas of infection such as sores and ulcers. Asiaticosides also stimulate the synthesis of lipids and proteins necessary for healthy skin. Finally centella strengthens veins by repairing the connective tissues surrounding veins and decreasing capillary fragility.

ACTIVE PROPERTIES

Centella has been found to have important healing effects on solid tissues, including skin, connective tissue, lymph tissues, blood vessels, and mucous membranes. Centella has found its most successful applications in treatment of conditions involving venous insufficiency, tissue inflammation and infection, and post-surgical healing.

DIRECTIONS FOR USE

50-100 mg/day internally. Topical applications available: 1% preparation twice/day.

HISTORICAL USES

- **Skin Injuries:** open wounds, sores, tears, cuts, ulcers, applied topically or taken internally
- **Confinement**: bed sores, phlebitis, tingling, nocturnal cramps
- **Venous Insufficiency**: phlebitis, varicose veins, cellulite, edema
- **Infections**: cellulitis, erysepilas, various other skin infections
- **Gynecology**: Pregnancy lesions, perineal lesion occurring during delivery and obstetric manipulations, radiation ulcers, episiotomy tears
- **Other**: sedative, tonic, learning, memory

COMMON NAME
Centella, gotu kola
LATIN NAME
Centella asiatica l.
ORIGIN
Madagascar (wild)
PART OF PLANT USED
Aerial part
ACTIVE SUBSTANCES
asiaticosides, triterpenes
STANDARD
10% asiaticosides

GOTU KOLA

(CENTELLA ASIATICA)

BIO-ENHANCING AGENTS:
bilberry, silicon, butcher's broom, zinc, vitamin C, E, D.

PROCESSING
Extraction with hydromethanolic or hydroacetonic solution.

TOXICITY, CAUTIONS & CONTRA-INDICATIONS
No known toxicity.

SCIENTIFIC REFERENCES
• Mowrey, D. (1990) Guaranteed Potency Herbs. A Compilation of writings on the subject.

ANALYSIS

Determination	
HPLC contents of total triterpenes calculated as asiaticoside	10.80%
Character	fine dark-green powder
Particle size	complies /micron (60 mesh)
Sulfated Ash	15.50%
Heavy Metals	complies ppm

GRAPE SEED EXTRACT

DESCRIPTION

Grape seed extract is a bioflavonoid-rich, potent extract which is used for fighting free radicals and maintaining capillary health. It is very similiar to pine bark extract, with a high content of proanthocyanidins (see active properties). Proanthocyanidins are found in many foods, but freezing, cooking and canning deactivate them. Sales of proanthocyanidins in France alone are $100 million per year.

PHARMACOLOGY

Free radicals do damage in the capillaries in two ways: (1) by inactivating a compound called a 1-antitripsin, whose role is to restrain the enzymes that break down collagen, elastin and hyaluronic acid, and (2) by turning the fats in the cell membranes rancid (lipid peroxidation). Proanthocyanidins protect both the 1-antitripsin and the lipids by neutralizing the specific types of free radicals most likely to damage them, and may also directly inhibit the damaging enzymes. Collagen, elastin and hyaluronic acid make up much of the inner wall and supporting matrix of the capillaries; when they are in good shape the capillaries stretch to let red blood cells through the tight places and do not let the fluids in the blood leak out. Proanthocyanidins have shown a marked tendency to accumulate in tissues with high contents of glycosaminoglycans (complex amino sugars), such as capillary walls and skin. This may also apply to cartilage and synovial fluid. Proanthocyanidins have also shown antimutagenic effects in vitro at high concentrations (250 mcg/ml).

ACTIVE PROPERTIES

Proanthocyanidins (also known as leucoanthocyanidins and pycnogenols) are a form of polyphenol, which is in turn a form of bioflavonoid. Proanthocyanidins are at least 15 to 25 times more powerful than vitamin E in neutralizing the iron and oxygen species free radicals that attack lipids.

HISTORICAL USES

Grape seed extract is used for its free radical fighting capabilities, and for a variety of conditions related to capillary health and permeability. It is synergistic with vitamin C– which is more potent and absorbed more rapidly when used together with Proanthocyanidins.

Proanthocyanidins have been indicated for:
- poor distribution of microcirculatory blood flow in the brain and heart;
- altered capillary fragility and permeability (in diabetes mellitus);
- chronic arterial/venous insufficiency in the extremeties;
- altered platelet aggregation and other characteristics of blood flow in capillaries;
- breakdown in the elastic fibers of the capillaries (collagen and elastin) due to free radical and enzyme action;
- microangiopathy of the retina, edema of the lymph nodes, varicose veins and other symptoms of the problems listed above;
- the cumulative effects of aging and reducing the risk of degenerative diseases.

COMMON NAME
Grape seed extract
LATIN NAME
Vitis vinifera
ORIGIN
Europe
PART OF PLANT USED
Seed
ACTIVE SUBSTANCES
Proanthocyanidins
STANDARD
95% polyphenols

GRAPE SEED EXTRACT

DIRECTIONS FOR USE

100 to 200 mg daily for 7 to 10 days, then 60 to 100 mg daily, or as desired. Usage ranges from 30 mg per day (venous-lymphatic insufficiency) to 300 mg per day (eye stress from use of video display terminal) in studies reporting significant results.

TOXICITY, CAUTIONS & CONTRA-INDICATIONS

Proanthocyanidins are almost completely non-toxic both in acute dosage (LD50>4,000mg/kg in rats & mice) and high long-term dosage (no toxic effects at 60 mg/kg/day for 12 months in dogs and 6 months in rats). They have no potential for causing mutations or birth defects, and have no adverse effect on fertility, pregnancy or nursing.

SCIENTIFIC REFERENCES

• Corbe, C., Boissin, J.P., & Siou, A., J. Fr. Ophtalmol, vol. 11, pg. 453, 1988.
• Doutremepuich, J.D., Barbier, A., & Lacheretz, F., Lymphology, vol. 24, pg. 135, 1991.
• Elstner, E.F., & Kleber, E., Flavonoids in biology and medicine, current issues in flavonoids research, National University of Singapore, Singapore, pp.227-235, 1990.
• Liviero, L., et al., International Symposium on Phytochemistry of Plants used in Traditional Medicine, 29 Sept. - 1 Oct., 1993, Lausanne.
• Groult, N., et al., Path. Biol., vol.39, pg. 277, 1991.

ANALYSIS

Determination	Results	Specification
Spectrophotometric contents of NaCl precipitates	39.3%	35.0 - 45.0%
Character: orange-rose powder	complies	complies
Solubility in water	complies	complies
Insoluble substances in water	0.4%	<=2.0%
TLC ID of cyanidol	complies	complies
UV ID	complies	complies
Particle size (200 mesh)	complies	<=70.0 microns
Procyanidolic value with reference to the anhydrous & solvent-free substance.	118.5	>=95.0
Sulphated Ash	0.43%	<=0.5%
Water (K. Fischer)	1.54%	<=8.0%
Heavy Metals	complies	<=10ppm
Iron	complies	<=20 ppm
Total residual organic solvents	0.05%	<=0.5%
Ethanol	0.04%	<=0.5%
Ethyl Acetate	0.01%	<=0.1%
Aceton	<0.005%	<=0.05%
Methylene chloride	<50.0 ppm	<=50.0 ppm
Other solvents	<50.0 ppm	<=50.0 ppm

GREEN TEA EXTRACT

DESCRIPTION
Green tea is natural dried leaves of the tea plant, Camellia sinensis. Black tea is oxidized green tea. Both have been used for thousands of years in Asia, as beverage and medicine. Green tea extract is a bioflavonoid-rich, potent extract which is used primarily for fighting free radicals. It has a high content of polyphenols, which are a class of bioflavonoids.

PHARMACOLOGY
The polyphenols in green tea are catechins, with multiple linked ring-like structures. Polyphenols are a form of bioflavonoids with several phenol groups. They control both taste and biological action. The dominant and most important catechin in green tea is (-) Epigallocatechin Gallate (EGCG), a potent antioxidant which is used for food production, as well as in animal research studies. The phenol groups capture pro-oxidants and free radicals. EGCG is over 200 times more powerful than vitamin E in neutralizing the pro-oxidants and free radicals that at-tack lipids in the brain, in vivo. It is 20 times more potent than vitamin E in reducing formation of perox-ides in lard by the Active Oxygen Method, in vitro.

ACTIVE PROPERTIES
Green tea extract is used primarily for its free radical fighting capa-bilities, but has a wide range of applications. Its key ingredient,(-) Epigallocatechin Gallate (EGCG), protects against digestive and res-piratory infections. (A solution of 1 mcg per ml of EGCG heavily inhibited influenza virus in vitro.) It helps block the cancer-promot-ing actions of carcinogens, ultra-violet light, and metastasis from an original site in the skin, stomach, small intestine, liver or lung. Higher quantities (0.5% to 1% of diet) were protective against high total and LDL-cholesterol levels on a cholesterol promoting diet in rats. Crude catechins at 0.5% of diet were effective in lowering blood pressures in spontaneously hypertensive rats. (Both EGCG and black tea catechins suppressed an-giotensin I converting enzyme,

HISTORICAL USES

- used primarily for its free radical fighting capabilities
- EGCG protects against digestive and respiratory infections
- helps block the cancer-promoting actions of carcinogens, ultraviolet light, and metastasis
- high total and LDL-cholesterol levels
- high blood pressure (suppresses angiotensin I converting enzyme)
- reduces platelet aggregation
- inhibiting pathogenic bacteria that cause food poisoning
- blocks the attachment of the bacteria associated with dental caries to the teeth

COMMON NAME
Green Tea
LATIN NAME
Camellia sinensis
ORIGIN
China and Japan, Asia
PART OF PLANT USED
leaf
ACTIVE SUBSTANCES
catechins, especially (-) Epigallocatechin Gallate (EGCG)
STANDARD
50% catechins (polyphenols)

GREEN TEA EXTRACT

which causes essential hypertension.) EGCG also reduces platelet aggregation about as much as aspirin or Ginkgo biloba extract. Green tea is very effective in inhibiting pathogenic bacteria that cause food poisoning, but increases levels of acidophilus (friendly) bacteria. 500 mg catechins (>= 250 mg EGCG) daily regularized bowel habits significantly. Green tea also blocks the attachment of the bacteria associated with dental caries to the teeth.

DIRECTIONS FOR USE
250 to 500 mg EGCG content daily, or as desired. Usage ranges from 250 mg to 2.5 g per day of EGCG content in studies reporting significant results.

BIO-ENHANCING AGENTS:
Catechins are synergistic with vitamins E and C, and with citric, malic and tartaric acids.

PROCESSING
Extraction with hydromethanolic or hydroacetonic solution.

TOXICITY, CAUTIONS & CONTRA-INDICATIONS
Green tea extract is non-toxic both in acute dosage and high long-term dosage (no significant effect on weight gain at 2% of the diet in 3 months in rats). It has no potential for causing mutations or birth defects, and has no adverse effect on fertility, pregnancy or nursing.

SCIENTIFIC REFERENCES
• Chem. Pharm. Bull., vol. 38, pg. 1049, 1990.
• Tohoku J. Exp. Med., vol. 166, pg. 475, 1992.
• Carcinogenesis, vol. 13, pp. 947 & 1491, 1992.
• Cancer Res., vol. 52, pp. 1162, 1943, 3875, 4050, 6657 & 6890, 1992.
• Cancer Lett., vol. 65, pg. 51, 1992.
• Muramatsu, K., Fukuyo, M., & Hara, Y., Effect of green Tea Catechin on Plasma Cholesterol Level in Cholesterol-Fed Rats, J. Nutr. Sci. Vitaminol., vol. 32, pp. 613-622, 1986.
• Sagasaka-Mitane, Y., Miwa, M., & Okada, S., Platelet Aggregation Inhibitors in Hot Water Extract of Green Tea, Chem. Pharm. Bull., vol. 38 (3), pp. 789-793, 1990.
• Horiba, N., et al., A Pilot Study of Japanese Green Tea as a Medicament: Antibacterial and Bactericidal Effects, Journal of Endodontics, vol. 17 (3), pp. 122-124, 1991.
• Hattori, M., et al., Chem. Pharm. Bull., vol. 38, pg. 717, 1990.

ANALYSIS

DETERMINATION	RESULTS
Description: fine light brown powder	Complies
Content: total Polyphenols	52.56%
Moisture	2.5%
Amino acid	<= 5 %
Ash	13.4%
Caffeine	8.0%
Lead	<60 mg/kg
Copper	<2 mg/kg
Microbiology	conforms

GUARANA

DESCRIPTION
Guarana is a caffeine-rich beverage from South America. Sometimes known as Brazilian Cocoa, guarana is made into a popular cola drink which is drunk in Brazil for energy and stimulation.

PHARMACOLOGY
Guarana is a natural stimulant due to its contents of xanthines. These xanthines include mainly guaranine (natural caffeine), theobromine, and theophylline. Guarana contains two to three times more caffeine than coffee or tea.

ACTIVE PROPERTIES
Guarana has been used as a stimulant, diuretic, and anti-diarrheic. Other applications have included as a nervine tonic, anti-fatigue stimulant, to reduce hunger, to relieve headaches and migraines, to alleviate PMS symptoms, and as an aphrodisiac.

PROCESSING
Guarana seeds are crushed and powdered. A hydroalcoholic extract is made.

DIRECTIONS FOR USE
50-100 mg./day

BIO-ENHANCING AGENTS
Yerba mate, coffee, tea, ginseng, gotu kola, kola nut

TOXICITY, CAUTIONS & CONTRA-INDICATIONS
Caffeine-containing substance. Do not overuse. Avoid during pregnancy. Dysuria is a common side-effect of guarana use.

SCIENTIFIC REFERENCES
- Mowrey, D. (1990) Guaranteed Potency Herbs. A Compilation of writings on the subject.
- Mowrey, D. (1986) The Scientific Validation of Herbal Medicine. Cormorant Books.

HISTORICAL USES

- For fatigue
- As a nervine tonic
- As a stimulant
- For diarrhea, gastrointestinal complaints
- For PMS symptoms; headaches, listlessness
- To quell hunger
- As an aphrodisiac
- As a systemic cleanser
- For neuralgia and other mild pains

ANALYSIS

Product	Paullinia cupana, Guarana
Type	Standardized Extract
Standardization	12.5 % total alkaloids
Loss on drying	5.35 %
Sulphated ash	3.6 %
pH	5.4
Heavy Metals	less than 100 ppm

COMMON NAME
Guarana, Uabano, Brazilian Cocoa, Brazilian Cola
LATIN NAME
Paullinia cupana
ORIGIN
Brazilian rain forests, South American countries
PART OF PLANT USED
seeds
ACTIVE SUBSTANCES
xanthines: guaranine (caffeine), theobromine, theophylline
STANDARD
12.5 % alkaloids

HAWTHORNE

DESCRIPTION
Hawthorne is a small thorny tree with white or red flowers and berries. Hawthorne is one of the most valuable cardiovascular tonics available.

PHARMACOLOGY
The berries are rich in flavonoids which have been shown to dilate peripheral and coronary blood vessels. This action helps alleviate hypertension and high blood pressure and reduce the severity and frequency of angina attacks. Hawthorne also is a rich source of procyanidins which have sedative and antispasmodic effects. The herb has also been shown to act as a cardiotonic, restoring both high and low blood pressure to normal. Hawthorne has been used in treating irregular heartbeats, spasms of the arteries (Raynaud's), and certain nervous disorders, such as insomnia.

PROCESSING
Dry, hydroalcoholic extract

DIRECTIONS FOR USE
250 mg/ day

BIO-ENHANCING AGENTS
valerian root, motherwort

TOXICITY, CAUTIONS & CONTRA-INDICATIONS
No known toxicity. May potentiate the action of digitalis.

SCIENTIFIC REFERENCES
- Mowrey, D. (1990) Guaranteed Potency Herbs. A Compilation of writings on the subject.
- Mowrey, D. (1986) The Scientific Validation of Herbal Medicine. Cormorant Books.
- Rewerski, W and Lewak, S. (1970) Hypotonic and sedative polyphenol and procyanidin extracts from hawthorn. Ger. Offen. 2:145-211.
- Ullsperger, R. (1951) Preliminary communication concerning a coronary vessel dilating principle from hawthorn. Pharmazie 6(4):141-144.

HISTORICAL USES

- Cardiotonic
- Angina
- Regular heartbeats
- Spasms in the arteries (Raynaud's syndrome)
- High and low blood pressure
- Old age vascular problems
- Hypertension
- Nervous disorders
- Insomnia
- Coronary artery and perfusion disorders
- Rhythmic disturbances / heart
- Aid digestion
- Dyspepsia and diarrhea

ANALYSIS

Product:	Crategus oxyacantha, Hawthorne Berries
Type	Standardized extract
Standardization	2% vitexin-2"-rhamnoside
Color	Brown powder
TLC identification of flavonoids	complies
pH	4.5-6.0
Ash	7 %
Heavy Metals	less than 100 ppm
Residual organic solvents	less than 0.2 %
Total aerobic microbial count	less than 1000 cfu/g

COMMON NAME
Hawthorne,
Mayblossom, whitethorn.

LATIN NAME
Crategus oxyacantha

ORIGIN
England, Europe, North America

PART OF PLANT USED
Berries

ACTIVE SUBSTANCES
flavonoid glycosides, saponins, procyanidins, trimethylamine, tannins.

STANDARD
2 % vitexin-2"-rhamnoside

HOPS

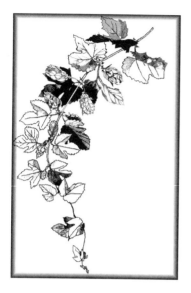

COMMON NAME
Hop, Hops

LATIN NAME
Humulus lupulus

ORIGIN
Netherlands, North American, Europe

PART OF PLANT USED
Female strobiles (fruit)

ACTIVE SUBSTANCES
Lupulin is comprised of the volatile oil and bitter resin. Volatile oil contains mainly humulene, myrcene, B-carophyllene, and farnescene. Bitter resin complex contains 2-Methyl-3-butonol, humulone, lumulone, lupulone, and valeronic acid. Other substances identified include tannins, flavonoid glycosides (rutin, quercetin, astragalin), and asparagine

STANDARD
5.2% alpha bitter acid or 2% essential oils

DESCRIPTION
Hops is a hedgerow climber with a tendency to twine around trees. Hops have been used since Roman times in brewing and as a traditional nervine and sedative herb. Hop tea has been recommended for insomnia, restlessness, and diarrhea. In addition, a hop pillow was frequently used in the past for the sedative effects of the volatile oils released while sleeping.

PHARMACOLOGY
Extensive modern research indicates that hops can relax smooth muscles as well as act as a sedative. The bitter acids, lupulone and humulone, are some of the identified active ingredients with sedative properties. The flavonglucosides have diuretic and spasmolytic properties. In addition estrogenic substances have been identified in hops and account for the traditional use of hops as an anaphrodisiac.

ACTIVE PROPERTIES
Hops has been used to treat digestive tract disorders involving spasms of the smooth muscle, especially irritable bowel syndrome and Crohn's disease.

PROCESSING
Ethanol extraction, type repercolation at room temperature. Evaporation at room temperature at reduced pressure. Spray drying with Maltodextrine as carrier substance.

DIRECTIONS FOR USE
100 mg/day

BIO-ENHANCING AGENTS
Valerian root, Skullcap, Passion Flower

HISTORICAL USES

- Insomnia
- Nervous Tension, restlessness
- As a sedative
- Hysteria
- Intestinal spasms, Crohn's Disease, Irritable Bowel Syndrome
- Inflammation
- As an anaphrodisiac
- Stimulate appetite
- Climacteric disorders
- Mild diuretic
- Increased breast milk for irritable infants

HOPS

TOXICITY, CAUTIONS & CONTRA-INDICATIONS

No known toxicity. Large quantities can have an anaphrodisiac effect. Female hop pickers have suffered from loss of menstruation from absorbing the oil through their hands. Hops are not recommended for persons suffering from depressive illness.

SCIENTIFIC REFERENCES

• Mowrey, D. (1990) Guaranteed Potency Herbs. A Compilation of writings on the subject.
• Mowrey, D. (1986) The Scientific Validation of Herbal Medicine. Cormorant Books.
• Wohlfart, R. et al. (1982) An investigation of sedative-hypnotic principles in Hops. Part 3. Plant Medica 45:224.
• Weiner, M. (1990) Weiner's Herbal. Mill Valley: Quantum Books.

ANALYSIS

Product	*Humulus lupulus*, Hops
Type	Standardized extract
Standardization	5.2% alpha-bitter acid
Color	Green powder with characteristic smell & taste
Loss on drying	<5%
TLC ID	extractives in 55% v/v ethanol
Heavy Metals	<5 ppm
Microbiology	
molds/yeasts	<100/g
coliforms	negative

HORSETAIL

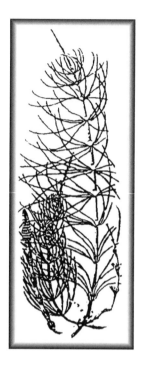

DESCRIPTION

Horsetail grass is a plant made up of bunches of leafless tubular stems or rushes. The plant grows in moist soil and concentrates minerals, particularly silica. The plant is also valued for its astringent and antibiotic properties. In folklore practices, horsetail grass was used to accelerate the healing of broken bones and connective tissue injuries and to promote healthy eyes, hair, skin and nails.

PHARMACOLOGY

The essential element, silicon, is present in very large amounts in horsetail grass. The element is present in the plant in its organic forms, silicon dioxide (SiO_2) or silicic acid/silicate ($Si(OH)_2$). Silica is essential for growth and healing, being a major constituent of bones, cartilage, connective tissue, and skin. In the body silica makes up part of the mucopolysaccharides (glycosaminoglycans) which play critical structural roles in bone and cartilage. The degeneration of tissues with age corresponds with decreasing levels of silica in the tissue. Silicic acid also stimulates an increase in white blood cells, helping to increase resistance to infection. In the past a tea of horsetail grass was frequently given to tuberculosis patients. The second major class of ingredients of horsetail grass is the saponins. These compounds have a mild diuretic effect. Horsetail is widely used for genitourinary problems including inflammations, kidney stones, enuresis, lithiasis, nephritis, gout, and prostate problems.

ACTIVE PROPERTIES

Besides the wound healing, connective tissue strengthening, and genitourinary properties, horsetail grass also possesses styptic properties, helping to heal bleeding ulcers. The plant has been used for arthritis and atherosclerosis since both joint and arterial tissue are rich in silica.

COMMON NAME
Horsetail Grass, Mare's Tail, Shave Grass, Joint Grass
LATIN NAME
Equisetum arvense
ORIGIN
Europe
PART OF PLANT USED
Herb (overground part)
ACTIVE SUBSTANCES
Silica, flavoglucosides, saponins (Equisetonin), alkaloids (nicotine, palustrine), manganese, magnesium, potassium, tannin.
STANDARD
10 % Silicic acid (7.87 silica)

HISTORICAL USES

- As a mild diuretic
- Broken nails, lifeless hair, hair loss, skin disorders
- Anemia
- General debilitation
- To stop bleeding
- For stomach ulcers
- Inflamed or enlarged prostate
- Cystitis, urinary stones
- Lung complaints
- Arteriosclerosis
- Pulmonary tuberculosis
- Strengthen immune system
- Shampoos and cosmetics

HORSETAIL

DIRECTIONS FOR USE
1.5 gm/day dried herb; 300 mg. extract

PROCESSING
Horsetail grass is gathered in early spring. The extract is prepared by water/ethanol repercolation at 20-30°C with the addition of sugars to increase the yield of silica. Evaporation at low temperature and pressure is then performed.

BIO-ENHANCING AGENTS
Echinacea, Chaparral, Parsley, Marshmallow, Slippery elm, Comfrey

TOXICITY, CAUTIONS & CONTRA-INDICATIONS
No known toxic effect for normal use. Avoid use with antihypertensive drugs, digitalis, corticosteroids, heparin, and lithium.

SCIENTIFIC REFERENCES
• Mowrey, D. (1990) Guaranteed Potency Herbs. A Compilation of writings on the subject.
• Mowrey, D. (1986) The Scientific Validation of Herbal Medicine. Cormorant Books.
• Sommer, L. et al. (1962) Antimicrobial activity of the volatile oil extracted from equisetum arvense. Farmacia Bucharest. 10:535.
• Weiner, M. (1990) Weiner's Herbal. Mill Valley: Quantum Books.

ANALYSIS

Type	Standardized extract
Standardization	7% silica
Character	corresponding
Loss on drying	2.9%
Ash	39.0%
Microbiological Content	
Microbiological Specifications (Pharm. Acta. Helv. 51(3):33-40. 1976)	
Gram negatives	absent
Escherichia coli	absent
Staphylococcus aureus	absent
Pseudomonas aeruginosa	absent
Salmonella sp.	absent

KAVA KAVA

DESCRIPTION
Kava Kava root has been used in the South Pacific for centuries as a relaxant herb. In this ethnobotanical format, the resinous juice is extracted from the root and made into a beverage. Kava is still widely used in South Pacific cultures. The Kava plants which are used in their native setting, and to make standardized extracts for use in Europe and the United States, have been selectively bred over many generations from wild cultivars that contain high levels of activity. Plants are reproduced from root stocks.

PHARMACOLOGY
Research into the source of Kava's activity has been going on for over 100 years. It is now widely accepted that the active compounds are a group of 15 lactones unique to the plant, and referred to as Kavalactones. There are also some alkaloids present, but it is not known whether or not these are responsible for any of Kava's activity. Kava's primary use is as a relaxant and sleep aid, and all researcheres discuss fondly its mildly psychoactive properties which induce a feeling of relaxation, peace, contentment and sharpening of the senses.

DIRECTIONS FOR USE
150-250 mg per cap/tab
Dosage: 1-3 caps/tabs

PROCESSING
Specific strains of Kava, with demonstrated high levels of activity are cultivated in plantations in the South Pacific, primarily Fiji. Extracts are made in Germany to meet OTC pharmaceutical standards.

BIO-ENHANCING AGENTS
Valerian root, Hops, Chamomile, Licorice

TOXICITY, CAUTIONS & CONTRA-INDICATIONS
None

SCIENTIFIC REFERENCES
• 'Kava: The Pacific Drug', Lebot, Merlin and Lindstrom. Yale University Press.

HISTORICAL USES

- Relaxant
- Sleep aid
- Headaches

ANALYSIS

Type	Standardized extract
Standardization	30.10% total Kavalactones
Character	yellow powder
Aerobic Plate	<10,000/g
E. coli	neg
Coliform	neg
Salmonella sp.	neg
Yeasts and Molds	<100/g

COMMON NAME
Kava Kava
LATIN NAME
Piper methysticum
ORIGIN
South Pacific Islands
PART OF PLANT USED
Dried root
ACTIVE SUBSTANCES
A group of lactones unique to the plant– Kavalactones
STANDARD
30% Kavalactones

KOLA NUT (COLA)

DESCRIPTION

Cola (also Kola and Cola Nut) is the seed kernel of a large African tree, Cola acuminata (P. Beauv.) Schott. & Endl. or Cola nitida Schott. & Endl., of the Sterculiaceae family, commercially grown around the world in the tropics as a caffeine stimulant. The nuts are basically round, 3/4" to 1 1/4" long, flattened and rounded on one side, irregularly scooped out on the other side, occuring in pairs. They start out white and turn a characteristic red or reddish gray when dried.

PHARMACOLOGY

Stimulant to the central nervous system, anti-depressive, astringent and diuretic. May relieve some migraine headaches. May have antioxidant activities due to its phenolic and anthrocyanin constituents.

ACTIVE PROPERTIES

Key constituents are caffeine, with traces of theobromine; tannins and phenolics, including d-catechin, l-epicatechin, kolatin, and kolanin (catechol and (-) epicatechol are lost on drying); phlobaphene; an anthocyanin pigment, kola red; betaine; protein; and starch.

TOXICITY, CAUTIONS & CONTRA-INDICATIONS

Not considered toxic. The 1901 text says, "Not infrequently, however, connected thought is rendered more difficult" as impressions become too fleeting. Do not use when caffeine is contraindicated.

DIRECTIONS FOR USE

Decoction: put 1-2 teaspoonfuls of [unextracted powder] in a cup of water, bring to boil and simmer gently for 10-15 minutes. Assuming a 4:1 concentration in extract, 1/4 to 1/2 teaspoon of extract would be equivalent, whether in capsule form or dissolved in a beverage.

COMMON NAME
Cola (also Kola and Cola Nut)

LATIN NAME
Cola acuminata (P. Beauv.) Schott. & Endl. or Colanitida Schott. & Endl.

ORIGIN
Tropics (originated in Africa)

PART OF PLANT USED
Seed kernel

ACTIVE SUBSTANCES
caffeine, with traces of theobromine; tannins and phenolics; an anthocyanin pigment, kola red

STANDARD
9.5% to 10.5% caffeine

HISTORICAL USES

- the capacity for physical exertion is augmented;
- ideas become clearer, thought flows more easily and rapidly, and fatigue and drowsiness disappear;
- increase power of enduring fatigue without food;
- comparable to guarana, teas, coffee, and other caffeine sources;
- act decisively in cardiac weakness;
- nervous debility, states of atony and weakness;
- nervous diarrhea, depression, anorexia, sea sickness;
- giving rise to euphoric states in some people;
- some varieties of migraine, but is unlikely to bring releif to those who regularly drink coffee or other caffeinated drinks;
- neurasthenia and hysteria, characterized by great mental despondency, foreboding, brooding, more of a quiet or silent character. It is especially indicated if the heart is feeble and irregular in its action, with general muscular feebleness.

KOLA NUT (COLA)

SCIENTIFIC REFERENCES
• Cushny, Arthur R., M.A., M.D., ABERD., A Textbook of Pharmacology & Therapeutics, 2nd edition, Lea Brothers and Co., Philadelphia & New York, 1901.
• U.S. Dispensatory, 19th. edition, pg. 1541, 1907.
• Hoffman, David, B. Sci. (Hons.), M. N. I. M. H., Therapeutic Herbalism, A Correspondence Course in Phytotherapy pg. 5-68.

ANALYSIS

Determination	Results	Specifications
Acidimetric contents of total alkaloids	10.5%	9.5-10.5%
Character: brown to reddish brown powder	complies	complies
TLC ID	complies	complies
pH (c=5, alcohol(50% v/v)	complies	complies
Loss on drying (T=105 C., t=14h)	5.4	5.0-7.0
Sulphated Ash	1.85%	<=5.0%
Heavy Metals	complies	<=100 ppm
Total Aerobic Microbial	<=1000 cfu/g	<=1000 cfu/g
Fungi	<=1000 cfu/g	<=1000 cfu/g
S. Aureus	absent	
Salmonella	absent	
E. coli	absent	
P. aeruginosa	absent	

LICORICE

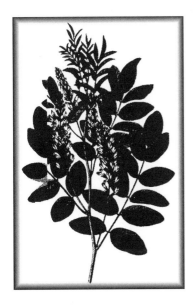

COMMON NAME
Licorice
LATIN NAME
Glycyrrhiza glabra
ORIGIN
Italy, Spain, Iran, Russia
PART OF PLANT USED
Roots
ACTIVE SUBSTANCES
glycyrrhizin, glycyrrhetinic acid, flavonoids, asparagine, iso-flavonoids, chalcones, coumarins, triterpenoid saponins.
STANDARD
(1) Deglycyrrhizinated licorice with 1-2% Glycyrrhizin
(2) 12% Glycyrrhizin

DESCRIPTION

Licorice has long been used for both culinary and medical purposes. Used for flavoring and sweetening candies and medical remedies, licorice also has potent effects of its own, particularly for ulcers and adrenal insufficiencies. Whole Licorice is used for cases of adrenal insufficiencies and inflammation. Another more widely used form is the deglycyrrhizinated one which is as effective as whole Licorice in its ulcer treating properties but without any hypertensive side effects.

PHARMACOLOGY

Licorice contains the glycoside, glycyrrhizin which has a similar structure and activity as the adrenal steroids. Licorice has an anti-inflammatory activity similar to cortisone and has been found useful for arthritis and allergies. In addition licorice has been used for mild Addison's disease and other adrenal insufficiencies, such as hypoglycemia. Licorice also acts like the hormone, ACTH, causing sodium retention, potassium depletion, and water retention. Excess consumption of licorice can lead to the classic symptoms of hyper-tension, with edema, increased blood pressure, potassium loss, and muscular weakness. Licorice is also highly effective in the treatment of gastrointestinal complaints, particularly peptic and gastric ulcers. The Deglycyrrhizinated form is most often used to avoid the hypertensive side effects of the glycyrrhetinic acid in whole Licorice. Licorice and DGL have a mild laxative effect and can protect the intestinal lining by increasing the production of mucus, thus alleviating heartburn and ulcers. Licorice and DGL also have a demulcent action and have been used for coughs and other bronchial complaints. Recent research has also revealed anti-bacterial, anti-toxin, and estrogenic effects for licorice.

DIRECTIONS FOR USE

600 mg/day DGL extract or 000 mg of regular extract 1/2 hour before meals.

BIO-ENHANCING AGENTS

Liver: milk thistle, dandelion, cascara, wild yam. *Stomach:* goldenseal, ginger, gentian root. *Adrenal Support:* panax ginseng, Siberian ginseng. *Arthritis:* alfalfa,

HISTORICAL USES

- Ulcers and stomach distress
- Inflammatory problems, arthritis
- Adrenal insufficiency, Addison's disease
- Hypoglycemia
- Cirrhosis and liver damage
- Skin problems, rashes, dermatitis, impetigo
- Coughs and bronchial complaints
- Bacterial infections
- Constipation
- As a female tonic

LICORICE

celery seed, chapparal. *Immune System:* echinacea, ginseng, Schisandra, saw palmetto. *Bronchial Complaints:* anise, yarrow, mullein.

TOXICITY, CAUTIONS & CONTRA-INDICATIONS

Glycyrrhetinic acid increases blood sodium and decreases potassium levels by stimulating renal tubules to absorb excessive amounts of water. Edema and slight rises in venous and arterial blood pressure may result. Potassium supplementation (75-100 mg.) prevents this problem. Persons with high blood pressure should supplement licorice root with potassium. Use of DGL form avoids this hypertensive effect.

SCIENTIFIC REFERENCES

• Mowrey, D. (1990) Guaranteed Potency Herbs. A Compilation of writings on the subject.
• Mowrey, D. (1986) The Scientific Validation of Herbal Medicine. Cormorant Books.
• Tagi, K. et al. (1965) Peptic ulcer inhibiting activity of licorice root. Proc. Int. Pharmacol. 7(1).
• Gaby, A. (1988) Deglycyrrhizinated licorice treatment of peptic ulcer. Townsend Letter for Doctors. July:306.

ANALYSIS

Product	*Deglycyrrhizinated Licorice*
Type	Standardized extract
Standardization	Deglycyrrhizinated with 1.5% glycyrrhizin
Loss on drying	4.1%
pH	5.6
Ash	14.1%
Storage	Sealed in cool, dry, dark place

MILK THISTLE

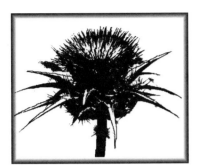

DESCRIPTION
Milk thistle was named Silybum by Dioscorides in 100 AD for its large purple thistle-like flower heads. Since ancient times, the plant was valued for its nutritional and medicinal properties. By the Middle Ages the seed of the Milk Thistle was commonly used to treat liver diseases, to promote the flow of bile, and as a general tonic for the stomach, spleen, gallbladder, female organs, and liver.

PHARMACOLOGY
Milk Thistle contains three potent liver protective flavonoids: silybin, silydianin, and silychristin, known collectively as silymarin. Numerous clinical trials have shown that silymarin and milk thistle extract can protect the liver. Silymarin counteracts the toxic effects of a wide variety of poisons, including alcohol, carbon tetrachloride, acetaminophen overdose, and the Deathcap mushroom, *Amanita phalloides* which causes death within a day. The mechanism of action of silymarin involves altering the membranes of hepatic cells to inhibit passage of toxins and increasing cellular regeneration by stimulating protein synthesis. Silymarin also has antioxidant activity and inhibits inflammatory enzymes. Recent research has indicated that silymarin helps to protect against depletion of the antioxidant glutathione in liver cells.

ACTIVE PROPERTIES
Milk Thistle extract has been the subject of numerous clinical trials and studies due to its potent liver protective properties. Milk thistle has been used for hepatitis, viral hepatitis, cirrhosis, jaundice, and fatty degeneration of the liver. Milk thistle has been used for indigestion since it promotes the flow of bile and thus helps emulsify fats. A positive therapeutic effect has been reported using silymarin for psoriasis. The Eclectics recommended milk thistle for varicose veins.

DIRECTIONS FOR USE
300-600 mg. /day.

COMMON NAME
Milk Thistle
LATIN NAME
Silybum marianum L. Gaertn. or *Carduus marianus L.*
ORIGIN
Northern America, Europe, moderate climates
PART OF PLANT USED
Seeds
ACTIVE SUBSTANCES
Flavonoids (silybin, silydianin, silychristin known collectively as Silymarin)
STANDARD
80% Silymarin

HISTORICAL USES

- Liver disease, acute, chronic hepatitis
- Protect liver from toxins, heavy metals, alcohol, poisons
- Cholagogue
- Fatty degeneration of the liver
- Jaundice
- Psoriasis
- Uterine tonic, menstrual difficulties
- Spleen, kidney, gall bladder tonic
- Varicose veins

MILK THISTLE

BIO-ENHANCING AGENTS

Dandelion root, turmeric, flavonoids, artichoke, schisandra

TOXICITY, CAUTIONS & CONTRA-INDICATIONS

No known toxicity, even in large doses.

PROCESSING

Milk thistle is harvested and extracted by methyl alcohol. The solution is filtered and evaporated under vacuum. The final defatted suspension is dried in a ventilation oven.

SCIENTIFIC REFERENCES

• Campos, R. et al. (1989) Silybin Dihemisuccinate protects against glutathione depletion and lipid peroxidation induced by acetaminophen on rat liver. Planta Medica. 55:417.
• Canini, F. et al. (1985) The use of silymarin in the treatment of alcoholic hepatic stenosis. Clin. Ther. 114:307.
• Ferenci, P. et al. (1989) Randomized controlled trial of silymarin treatment in patients with cirrhosis of the liver. J. Hepat. 9:105.
• Hruby, C. (1984) Silibinin in the treatment of Deathcap Fungus poisoning. Forum 6:23.
• Koch, HP et al. (1985) Silymarin: Potent inhibitor of cyclic AMP phosphodiesterase. Meth. Find. Espt. Clin Pharm. 7:409.
• Mowrey, D. (1990) Guaranteed Potency Herbs. A Compilation of writings on the subject.
• Mowrey, D. (1986) The Scientific Validation of Herbal Medicine. Cormorant Books.
• Weiner, M. (1990) Weiner's Herbal. Mill Valley: Quantum Books.

ANALYSIS

Product	Milk Thistle
Type	Standardized extract
Standardization	84.50% based on Silibin
Character	light yellow powder
Ash	0.25% (<0.5%)
TLC ID	complies
Microbiology: Total Aerobic Count	<1,000/g
Fungi	>100/g
Pathogenic Bacteria	none
Heavy Metals	>10 ppm
Pesticides	none

NETTLES

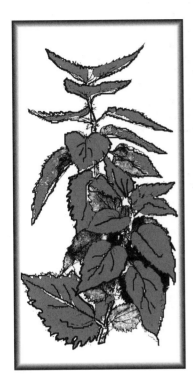

COMMON NAME
Nettles, Stinging Nettles
LATIN NAME
Urtica dioica
ORIGIN
Europe, Israel
PART OF PLANT USED
Leaves of young plants
ACTIVE SUBSTANCES
formic acid, histamine, acetylcholine, 5-hydroxytryptamine, glucoquinones, chlorophyll, minerals (iron, magnesium, silica, potassium, sulphur), vitamins A, C, B2, and B5, chlorophyll.
STANDARD
1-2% plant silica

DESCRIPTION

Stinging nettles grow throughout the world. Their name is derived from the presence of stinging hairs on their leaves and stems which when touched inject formic acid and histamine into the skin and cause urticaria, (or irritation and inflammation). Nettles have been widely used as food, medicine, cosmetics, and clothing.

PHARMACOLOGY

Nettles are a rich source of trace elements, absorbing and accumulating them. Nettles contain formic acid and the neurotransmitters acetylcholine, 5-hydroxy tryptamine, and histamine which are responsible for the sting. These constituents are thought to endow nettles with their anti-arthritic and anti-rheumatic and expectorant properties.

ACTIVE PROPERTIES

Because of their rich nutritional content, nettles have traditionally been given to anemic, exhausted, debilitated or recuperating people as soups or teas. The stinging properties are lost when the plant is cooked. Nettles also have been traditionally used as an important hair and skin tonic. The high quantity of silicon has made nettles highly useful in stimulating hair growth, improving the condition of the hair and skin and treating dandruff. Nettles have been used internally and externally to treat eczema. Nettle juice has been used as an astringent or styptic to stop bleeding and to treat wounds.

The best known use of nettles is in the treatment of gout and other rheumatic conditions. A decoction of the leaves or the expressed juice has been shown to mobilize uric acid from the joints and eliminate it through the kidneys.

Recently a randomized, double-blind, clinical trial has shown the usefulness of nettles in the treatment of allergic rhinitis or hayfever.

HISTORICAL USES

- Gout
- Arthritis, tendonitis, sciatica, lumbago
- Eczema
- Hair loss and deterioration
- Allergic rhinitis, hayfever, sinusitis, sinus congestion
- Anemia, exhaustion, recovery
- Astringent, Styptic, wound healing
- Profuse menstruation
- Benign prostatic hypertrophy
- Anti-inflammatory
- Mild diuretic
- Encourage lactation
- Lower blood sugar

NETTLES

PROCESSING
Only the young top leaves are harvested from plants grown in clean uncontaminated areas. Extraction uses only water and alcohol, similar to traditional methods. The extract is concentrated to a paste, prepared as a liposoluble liquid extract for cosmetic use or spray dried to produce a stable pure powder.

DIRECTIONS FOR USE
750 mg extract /day

TOXICITY, CAUTIONS & CONTRA-INDICATIONS
No known toxicity.

SCIENTIFIC REFERENCES
• Krstic-Pavlovic, N. and Dzamic, R. (1985) Astringent and mineral components in the leaves of nettle (Urtica dioica, L.) from many natural locations. Agrochemija. 1985:191-198.
• Smith, T.A. (1977) Tryptamine and related compounds in plants. Phytochemistry. 16:171.
• Caceres, A. et al. (1987) Diuretic activity of plants used for the treatment of urinary ailments in Guatemala. J. Ethnopharmaco. 19:233-245.
• Baraibar, C. et al. (1983) Acute and chronic toxicity studies on Nettle (Urtica dioica, L.). An. Bromatol. 35:99-103.
• Mittman, P. (1990) Randomized, Double-Blind study of freeze-dried Urtica Dioica in the treatment of allergic rhinitis. Planta Medica 56:44-47.

ANALYSIS

Type	Standardized extract
Standardization	1.6% Silica
Taste	Conforms
Loss on drying	2.17%
pH	7.08
Ash	39.61%
Bulk density -packed	0.72
-loose	0.61
Heavy Metals	conforms
Microbiology	
Total count per gram	1000
Coliforms	<10
E. coli	<10
Staph aureus	neg
salmonella	neg
yeasts and molds	<20
Storage	

PASSION FLOWER

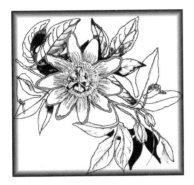

DESCRIPTION
Passion flower is a woody vine with flowers which reminded early Jesuit travelers of the passion or suffering of Christ. The plant produces a small berrylike fruit called granadilla or water lemon.

PHARMACOLOGY
Passion Flower contains glycosides (containing alkaloids) and flavonoids. Low levels of serotonin have been identified which may help explain the use of passion flower as a natural calmative, mood shifter and aid to concentration. Another compound called maltol has been shown to have mild sedative properties. The harmane alkaloids have been shown to be spasmolytic toward smooth muscle and to lower blood pressure by expanding heart coronary vessels.

ACTIVE PROPERTIES
For the past 200 years passion flower has been used to tranquilize and settle edgy nerves. Passion flower induces sleep without causing confusion upon awakening. Passion flower has been used by women to calm nerves and induce relaxation during the periods of hormonal adjustment found during menses, parturition, and menopause.

PROCESSING
Dried aerial parts are gathered during fruiting season. A dry hydroalcoholic extract is made.

DIRECTIONS FOR USE
100-200 mg/day

BIO-ENHANCING AGENTS
Hops, chamomile, skullcap, wood betony, valerian, L-tryptophan, GABA

COMMON NAME
Passion Flower
LATIN NAME
Passiflora incarnata
ORIGIN
North America, Europe, South America
PART OF PLANT USED
Dried aerial parts, gathered during fruiting season
ACTIVE SUBSTANCES
glycosides, flavonoids, harmine and harmane alkaloids (passiflorine, aribine, loturine, yageine), maltol
STANDARD
3.5-4.0 % isovitexin (flavonoids)

HISTORICAL USES

- Mild sedative
- Sleeplessness
- Nervous and high strung children, hyperactivity
- Cardiovascular neuroses
- Concentration problems
- Hormonal adjustment, menses, parturition, menopausal problems
- Bronchial asthma
- Hemorrhoidal inflammations
- Antispasmodic
- Analgesic
- Anti-convulsant

PASSION FLOWER

TOXICITY, CAUTIONS & CONTRA-INDICATIONS

No known toxicity. Use standardized whole plant extracts.

SCIENTIFIC REFERENCES

• Mowrey, D. (1990) Guaranteed Potency Herbs. A Compilation of writings on the subject.
• Mowrey, D. (1986) The Scientific Validation of Herbal Medicine. Cormorant Books.
• Weiner, M. (1990) Weiner's Herbal. Mill Valley: Quantum Books.
• Lutomski, J. et al. (1981) The meaning of Passion Flower in the healing arts. Pharmazie in Unserer Zeit. 10(2):45-49.

ANALYSIS

Product:	Passion Flower
Type	Standardized extract
Standardization	3.54% (3.5 -4.0%)
Characteristic	light brown amorphous powder
Solubility	
in water (c=2)	complies: clear or opalescent solution
in alcohol (50% v/v)(c=2)	complies: clear or opalescent solution
pH	4.0 (4.0-6.0)
Ash	17.6% (<=20.0)
Heavy Metals	<100.0 (<100.0 ppm)
Total residual organic solvents	0.01% (<=0.05%)
Ethanol	<0.005 (<=0.5%)
Methanol	0.01% (<=0.05%)
Methylene chloride	<0.005% (<=0.005%)
other	<0.005% (<=0.005%)
Microbiological content	
fungi	<100.0 (<=100.0) cfu/g
staph aureus, salmonella	absent
E. coli	absent

PYGEUM

COMMON NAME
Pygeum, African Pygeum
LATIN NAME
*Pygeum africanum or Prunus
africana*
ORIGIN
Southern Africa, Madagascar,
Central Africa
PART OF PLANT USED
Bark
ACTIVE SUBSTANCES
Phytosterols (sitosterols),
Pentacyclic triterpenoids, feru-
lic esters of long-chain fatty
alcohols
STANDARD
12% phytosterols (beta-sito-
sterol)

DESCRIPTION

Pygeum is a large evergreen tree, growing in the higher plateaus of southern Africa. Traditionally the bark of the tree was collected and powdered, then drunk as a tea for genito-urinary complaints. Recently numerous clinical trials have demonstrated the usefulness of a standardized extract of pygeum for prostatic hyperplasia, particularly benign prostatic hypertrophy (BPH).

PHARMACOLOGY

Pygeum contains three groups of active components: Phytosterols such as beta-sitosterol; pentacyclic triterpenoids, such as ursolic and oleanic acids; and ferulic esters of fatty alcohols, particularly the ferulic esters of docosanol and tetracosanol. The phytosterols, particularly beta-sitosterol are found in numerous plants and are anti-inflammatory, inhibiting the synthesis of prostaglandins. Beta-sitosterol has been shown to be useful in cases of BPH by helping to reduce the normally elevated levels of prostaglandins in these patients. The elimination of the excess blood and vasal congestion helps reduce the size of prostate adenomas. The pentacyclic triterpenoids also help inhibit inflammation by blocking enzymatic activity. They are effective anti-edema agents and also help increase the integrity of small veins and capillaries. The third active group, the ferulic esters of long-chain fatty acids, act by inhibiting the absorption and metabolism of cholesterol. BPH and other cases of enlarged prostates are characterized by containing abnormally high levels of cholesterol.

ACTIVE PROPERTIES

Pygeum has been studied in numerous double-blind clinical trials and found to be effective in treating a wide range of prostatic hyperplasis. Efficacy was determined by measuring the effects of extracts of pygeum on numerous parameters, including dysuria, nycturia, frequent urination, abdominal heaviness, residual urine,

HISTORICAL USES

Reported to be of benefit in:
• Prostatitis
• Benign Prostatic Hypertrophy (BPH)
• Urine retention
• Incontinence
• Polyuria or frequent urination
• Dysuria
• Stangury or painful urination
• Nycturia or nocturia (nocturnal urination)
• Cancer of the prostate
• Adenomatous fibrosclerosis

PYGEUM

voiding volume, prostate volume, and peak flow. Consumption of pygeum extract resulted in significant amelioration of symptoms, reduction in prostate size, and clearance of bladder neck urethral obstruction.

DIRECTIONS FOR USE
100-200 mg extract / day in divided quantities for several months.

BIO-ENHANCING AGENTS
Saw Palmetto

TOXICITY, CAUTIONS & CONTRA-INDICATIONS
No toxicity reported in the clinical trials.

PROCESSING
Air dried bark from the trunk of Pygeum africanum is passed through a screen and extracted with chloroform to isolate the fat-soluble fractions. The lipophilic extracts are filtered and concentrated to dryness under vacuum until complete elimination of chlorinated solvent.

ANALYSIS

Product	Pygeum
Type	Standardized extract
Standardization	12.36% Beta sitosterol
Character	brown soft mass
Loss on drying	1.05%
Ash	0.35%
Heavy Metals	complies
Microbiological Specifications	
Gram negatives	absent
E. coli	absent
Staph. aureus	absent
Pseudomonas aeruginosa	absent
Salmonella sp.	absent

SCIENTIFIC REFERENCES
• Bassi, P. et al. (1987) Standardized extract of Pygeum africanum in the treatment of benign prostate hypertrophy. Minerva Urologica 39:45.
• Marcoli, M. et al. (1985) New trends in Andro. Sci. 1:39.
• Mowrey, D. (1990) Guaranteed Potency Herbs. A compilation of writings on the subject.
• Thieblot, L. et al. (1971) Action preventive d'un extrait d'ecorce de plante africaine "Pygeum africanum" sur l'adenome prostatique experimental chez le rat. (Preventative action of an African plant extract, "Pygeum africanum" on experimental prostate adenoma in the rat) Therapie 26:575.
• Zurita, E.L. et al (1984) Treatment of prostatic hypertrophy with extract African prunus. Rev. Bras. Med. 41:48.

REISHI MUSHROOM EXTRACT

COMMON NAME
Reishi, also ling chih, ling chih mushroom, ling-zhi, mannentake

LATIN NAME
Ganoderma lucidum

ORIGIN
British Columbia (cultivated), also China, Japan

PART OF PLANT USED
whole fruiting body (mushroom)

ACTIVE SUBSTANCES
ganoderic acids (triterpenes), polysaccharides, ergosterols

STANDARD
Triterpenes: >= 4 % by HPLC
Polysacharides: >= 10 % by phenol-sulphuric method and photospectrometer.

DESCRIPTION
Reishi (Ganoderma lucidum (Leyss. ex Fr.) P. Karst) is also known as Ganoderma in the U.S. and Canada. It is called Ling-zhi or "mushroom of immortality" in China; and Reishi or Mannentake, "10,000 year-old mushroom" in Japan. Reishi is a basidomycetes, or polypore (with pores under the cap, instead of gills) that grows on the trunks or stumps of trees. Prune trees result in the highest levels of ganoderic acid. Although it typically has a kidney-shaped cap form on a slightly twisted columnar stalk, it also can look like deer antlers and many other shapes. It is distinguished by brownish-red color with almost-black and orange stripes, which are also highly variable.

PHARMACOLOGY
The proteins contain all of the essential amino acids, and most commonly occurring non-essential amino acids and amides. The fatty acids are largely unsaturated, and reishi are rich in vitamins (especially B3, B5, C & D) and minerals (especially calcium, phosphorus & iron). Reishi has the most active polysaccharides (long chains of sugars) among medicinal plant sources. Reishi is the only known source of a group of triterpenoides known as ganoderic acids, which have a molecular structure similar to steroid hormones. A study of nine edible medicinal mushrooms connected antitumor activity to polysaccharides and fatty substances that were probably ergosterols. Reishi also neutralized free radicals such as carbon tetrachloride and ethionine in animal livers, and reversed fatty infiltration.

INDICATIONS
Cancer, side-effects of cancer treatments including radiation, chemotherapy and surgery, high altitude stress, high cholesterol and hyperlipidemia, high blood pressure, chronic (post-viral) fatigue syndrome and AIDS, weaknesses of the lung, wasting symdromes, spiritual malaise, difficulty concentrating, poor digestion, insomnia, and poorly regulated immune response. Reishi is in the most highly rated category of herbs ("Superior"), in terms of multiple benefits and lack of side effects, in Traditional Chinese Medicine.

ACTIVE PROPERTIES
The polysaccharides and ergosterols probably work together to stimulate natural immune functions that tend to be suppressed by cancers and immune disorders. Ganoderic acids are responsible for the anti-allergy effects and improved oxygen utilization. Reishi greatly reduced the symptoms (headaches, nausea, vomiting, insomnia, heart palpitations and extreme fatigue) of oxygen deprivation among Chinese workers who traveled to the high plateau of Tibet, climbing 15,000 feet in 3 days in the process. Reishi is also effective in reducing the symptoms of cardiovascular blockage and disease, including angina, palpitation,

HISTORICAL USES

- Cancer (side effects of cancer treatments including radiation, chemotherapy and surgery)
- high altitude stress
- high cholesterol and hyperlipidemia
- high blood pressure
- chronic (post-viral) fatigue syndrome and AIDS
- weaknesses of the lung
- wasting syndromes
- spiritual malaise
- difficulty concentrating
- poor digestion
- insomnia
- poorly regulated immune response.

REISHI MUSHROOM EXTRACT

(continued from Active Properties)

fullness in the chest, dizziness and headache, shortness of breath, insomnia and weariness, and loss of memory in 65% or more of the patients in various studies. Reishi is a true adaptogen, enhancing health and normal functions of the body. For example, while it increases some components of immune response for cancer patients, it also inhibits pathological immune functions in auto-immune diseases such as myasthenia gravis. It has been reported to reduce the histamine release associated with allergic reactions, and help prevent anaphylactic reaction. It also increased immunoglobulin A levels in 2,000 chronic bronchitis patients.

DIRECTIONS FOR USE

For general tonification and protection, 150 to 350 mg or more of a 10:1 (10 g dried Reishi makes 1 g extract) or stronger extract daily, between meals. If digestive upset is experienced, take with meals. Estimate for therapeutic use in severe conditions: 3 to 9 grams extract divided into three doses, daily for several months, then taper back to 1 to 6 grams daily if desired, or as recommended by a health care practitioner. For high blood pressure, 750 mg twice daily (10:1). Initial results may take a week to develop, and maximum benefits may take 2 weeks or more.

BIO-ENHANCING AGENTS

Take 500 to 1000 mg vitamin C with each dose of Reishi to increase absorption. Also accompanying Reishi with astragalus, ginseng, salvia, echinacea, beta carotene, St. John's wort, and/or skullcap, as appropriate, is recommended for maximum results.

TOXICITY, CAUTIONS & CONTRA-INDICATIONS

None. High doses of unextracted powder may lead to loosening of the stools, dry mouth, skin rash, or slight digestive upset initially (extracts can be designed to reduce this).

PROCESSING

Cultivated on solid wood logs. Mushrooms chopped, cooked in alcohol & water at 75 C. for 3 hours. Solids separated and cooked again. Solids centrifuged off and liquids filtered to clarify. Liquids concentrated under vacuum at 60 C. Concentrate spray dried (no carrier). Final concentration is 12 to 15 pounds dry mushroom to 1 pound extract, in a fine, dry, reddish brown powder.

SCIENTIFIC REFERENCES

• Dharmananda,S., Medicinal Mushrooms, Bestways Magazine, July 1988
• Kohda, H., et al., The biologically active constituents of Ganoderma lucidum, Chem. Pharm. Bull., vol. 33 (4), pp. 1367-1374, 1985.
• Nishitoba, T., et al., Novel Triterpenoids and a Steroid from the Fungus Ganoderma lucidum, Agric. Biol. Chem., vol. 52 (1), pp. 211-216, 1988.
• Sone, Y., et. al., Structures and Antitumor Activities of the Polysaccharides Isolated from Fruiting Body and the Growing Culture of Mycelium of Ganoderma lucidum, Agric. Biol. Chem., vol. 49 (9), pp. 2641-2653, 1985.
• Tsung, P. K., Anticancer and Immunostimulating Polysaccharides, Oriental Healing Arts Bulletin, vol. 12 (1), pp. 1-10, 1987.
• Yamada, H., The Structure and Pharmacological Activity of Polysaccharides in Sino-Japanese Medicine, Oriental Healing Arts Bulletin, vol. 12 (1), pp. 11-23, 1987.
• Research Group of Hunan Institute of Pharmaceutical Industry, A Spot Survey on the Prevention of Acute Unadapted Symptoms At Plateau with Ganoderma, Chinese Traditional and Herbal Drugs, vol. 6, pp. 29-31, 1987.
• Third Hospital of Hong Qiao district of Tianjin, Clinical Observation of Hyperlipidemia Treated with Ganoderma Tablets, Chinese Traditional and Herbal Drugs, vol. 1, pp. 35-37, 1977.
• Nanjing Branch of the National Medical Society, Clinical Observation on the Treatment of 103 Cases of Coronary Heart Disease with Ganoderma Shu Xin Tablets, Chinese Traditional and Herbal Drugs, vol. 6, pp. 32-33, 1987.
• Jones, Kenneth, Reishi: Ancient Herb for Modern Times, Sylvan Press, Issaquah, Wash., 1991.

ANALYSIS

Standardization	4% Triterpenes, 10.0% Polysaccharides
Moisture	4.8 %
Protein	23.6 %
Lipids	6.1 %
Carbohydrates	45.1 %
Ash	20.4 %
Minerals (mg / gm)	
Phosphorus	78.7
Potassium	43.1
Magnesium	9.08
Heavy Metals (mcg / gm)	
Lead	5.0
Cadmium	nd (none detected)
Arsenic	nd
Mercury	nd
Microbiological	
Total plate count	<= 7,000 CFU / gram
Total coliform	negative
Pesticides	negative for Organochlorines

SAW PALMETTO

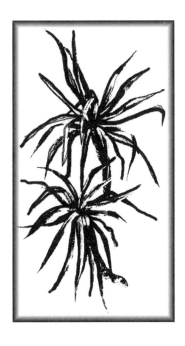

COMMON NAME
Saw Palmetto, Sabal
LATIN NAME
Serenoa serrulata, Seronoa repens, Sabal serulata
ORIGIN
North American Atlantic Coast
PART OF PLANT USED
Berries
ACTIVE SUBSTANCES
steroidal saponins, fatty acids, phytosterols, volatile oil, resin, tannins
STANDARD
90% free fatty acids

DESCRIPTION
Saw Palmetto is a small palm tree with large leaves and large deep red-blackberries. The berries were used by the American Indians as a general tonic to nourish the body and encourage appetite and normal weight gain. The berries were also used in the treatment of genito-urinary tract problems including enuresis, nocturia, and urinary tract disorders. Recent clinical trials have shown that saw palmetto berries are helpful in the treatment of benign prostatic hyperplasia.

PHARMACOLOGY
Saw Palmetto berries contain an oil with a variety of fatty acids and phytosterols. These fatty acids include capric, caprylic, caproic, lauric, palmitic, and oleic acid and their ethyl esters. The major phytosterols are beta-sitosterol, stigmasterol, cycloartenol, stigmasterol, cycloartenol, lupeol, lupenone, and 24-methyl-cycloartenol. The fat soluble extract of saw palmetto berries has been shown to inhibit the conversion of testosterone (DHT) which is thought to be responsible for the enlargement of the prostate. In addition saw palmetto extract inhibits the binding of DHT to receptors thus blocking DHT's action and promoting the breakdown of the potent compound.

ACTIVE PROPERTIES
The North American Indians used saw palmetto berries as a remedy for atrophy of the testes, impotence, inflammation of the prostate, and low libido in men. The berries are also recommended for infertility, painful periods, and lactation in women. The berries also have a traditional use as a tonic and expectorant for mucous membranes, particularly the bronchial passages.

HISTORICAL USES

- Urinary tract disorders, nocturia, enuresis
- Benign Prostatic Hypertrophy, prostate inflammation
- Impotence, low libido
- Atrophy of the testes
- Infertility in women
- Increase lactation
- Painful periods, tonic for ovarian function
- Expectorant, inhalant, bronchitis, asthma, catarrh, colds
- General nutritional tonic to increase fat, muscle, strength
- Tonic for mucous membranes
- Mildly sedative to the nervous system
- Anti-inflammatory
- Appetite stimulant, improve digestion
- Thyroid deficiency

SAW PALMETTO

DIRECTIONS FOR USE
320 mg / day

BIO-ENHANCING AGENTS
African Pygeum

**TOXICITY, CAUTIONS &
CONTRA-INDICATIONS**
No reported toxicity.

PROCESSING
Purified fat soluble extract.

SCIENTIFIC REFERENCES
• Campault, G. et al. (1984) A double blind trial of an extract of the plant Seronoa repens in benign prostatic hyperplasia. Br. J. Clin Pharm. 18:461.
• Mowrey, D. (1986) The Scientific Validation of Herbal Medicine. Cormorant Books.

ANALYSIS

Product	Saw Palmetto
Type	Standardized extract
Standardization	90% free fatty acids
Character	yellow color
Solubility	soluble in hexane
Loss on drying	5.5%
Assay: Main free fatty acids	
Caprylic acid	.7%
Capric acid	.6%
Lauric acid	19.3%
Myristic acid	12.4%
Palmitic acid	8.1%
Palmitoleic acid	.3%
Stearic acid	1.9%
Oleic acid	41.2%
Linoleic acid	2.3%
Linolenic acid	0.9%
Arachidic acid	0.04%
Main Esters of:	
Caprylic acid	.12%
Capric acid	.4%
Lauric acid	2.3%
Myristic acid	0.6%
Palmitic acid	0.4%
Oleic acid	1.7%
Linoleic acid	0.6%
Acid value	148.6
Saponification value	222.2
Iodine value	42.5
Unsaponifiable value	1.7%
Sterols	1.4%
Microbiological Specifications	
Gram negatives	absent
E. coli	absent
Staph. aureus	absent
Pseudomonas aeruginosa	absent
Salmonella sp.	absent

SCHISANDRA

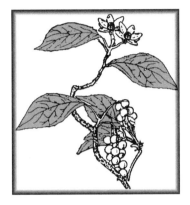

DESCRIPTION
Schisandra has been used in folk medicine throughout the ages, particularly in China and Tibet. The plant is a creeping vine with small red berries. In hunting and gathering tribes, the dried red berries sustained tribes in Northern China. Schisandra has been classified as an adaptogen, helping to regulate and normalize the functions of the body and help increase resistance to stress. The Chinese name, Wu wei tzu, (meaning five flavored seeds) refers to the five major tastes of the fruit: sweet, sour, pungent, bitter, and salty which correspond with the five elemental phases of Oriental Medicine.

PHARMACOLOGY
Schisandra contains various lignans, mainly schisandrins. These lignans have been found to prevent liver damage, stimulate liver repair, and stimulate normal liver functioning. These properties appear to be related to the antioxidant abilities of the various schisandrins. Schisandra further helps in digestion, regulating gastric acid release. Other studies have shown that extracts of Schisandra are stimulating to the CNS and are cholinergic. There have been numerous reports on Schisandra's ability to quicken reflexes, increase work efficiency, control anger, combat neurasthenias (headaches, insomnia, dizziness, palpitations). Other reports have mentioned increased cognitive function and increased memory. And a recent study concluded that Schisandra may be a useful agent to reverse depression, particularly that due to adrenergic exhaustion.

ACTIVE PROPERTIES
Recent research studies have indicated that Schisandra has numerous biological activities, including: antibacterial, mild stimulant, liver protective, antidepressant, antioxidant, antitoxin, adaptogen, and cardiotonic. In Oriental Medicine, Schisandra is recommended

COMMON NAME
Schisandra;
Chinese Wu wei tzu; Japanese Gomishi; Korean Omicha
LATIN NAME
Schisandra chinensis
ORIGIN
China
PART OF PLANT USED
Fruit, seeds
ACTIVE SUBSTANCES
Lignans (Schisandrins, Gomisin A) B-bisabolene, vitamin C, E
STANDARD
9% Schisandrins

HISTORICAL USES

- Endurance, Increased resistance to stress
- As an adaptogen
- Liver, kidney, lung tonic
- Anti-bacterial
- Anti-oxidant
- Anti-toxin
- Liver protective, liver stimulant, liver diseases
- Digestion promoter
- Aphrodisiac (male staying power, female libido)
- Hypoxia, high altitude sickness
- Depression
- Neurasthenia (headaches, dizziness, insomnia, palpitations)
- Increased cognitive functions, increased memory
- Anti-convulsant
- Increased reflexes
- Visual fatigue, near-sightedness, astigmatism

SCHISANDRA

for the lungs, liver and kidneys, including as an aphrodisiac (kidney element). Schisandra is also a registered medicine in Russia for vision problems since the herb has been found to prevent eye fatigue and increase acuity.

PROCESSING
Percolation / organic solvent at a low temperature and over a long time. Evaporation at low temperature and pressure.

DIRECTIONS FOR USE
100 mg. / twice day extract

BIO-ENHANCING AGENTS
Milk Thistle Extract, Dandelion.

TOXICITY, CAUTIONS & CONTRAINDICATIONS
No known toxicity. Should be avoided by persons with peptic ulcers, epilepsy, high blood pressure. Should not be used during pregnancy except to promote uterine contractions during labor.

SCIENTIFIC REFERENCES
• Ahumada F. Et al (1989) Studies on the effect of Schisandra chinensis extract on horses submitted to exercise and maximum effort. Phytotherapy Res. 3(5):175.
• Hancke, J. et al (1986) Antidepressant activity of selected natural products. Planta Medica 6:542.
• Hikino, H. et al (1984) Anti-hepatotoxic actions of lignoids from Schisandra chinensis fruits. Planta Medica 50(3):213.
• Mowrey, D. (1992) Schisandra: The Five Elemental Energies. Guranteed Potency Herbs: Next Generation Herbal Medicine, Vol. II.
• Mowrey, D. (1990) Guranteed Potency Herbs: A compilation of writings on the subject.
• Wahlstrom, M. (1987) Adaptogens. Utgivare, Goteborg.
• Weiner, M. (1990) Weiner's Herbal. Mill Valley: Quantum Books.

ANALYSIS

Product	Schisandra
Type	Standardized extract
Standardization	9% Schisandrins
Character	red-brown fine powder
Particle size	100% through 40 mesh
Ash	2.0% -2.5%
Loss on Drying	2.64%
Microbiological Content	<1000.0 / g
Aerobic plate	<10,000/g
E.coli	neg
Coliform	neg
Yeasts and Molds	<100/g
Salmonella	neg

SHIITAKE MYCELIA EXTRACT

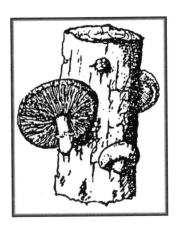

COMMON NAME
Shiitake Mycelia extract, lentinus edodes mycelia extract
LATIN NAME
Lentinus edodes
ORIGIN
British Columbia (originally Japan, Asia)
PART OF PLANT USED
Mycelia
ACTIVE SUBSTANCES
a new peptidomannan, KS-2 a water solubilized lignin derivative, EPS-3
STANDARD
3.2% KS-2

DESCRIPTION
The Shiitake mushroom (Lentinus edodes) grows on the trunks or stumps of trees. The mycelia of shiitake is the immature growing stage of the shiitake lifecycle. t grows as long threads, and absorbs and transforms lignans and other nutrients in the wood or culture medium it is growing in, before creating the fruiting body we think of as a mushroom. The shiitake mycelial extract is a fine brown, whitish brown, or tan powder.

PHARMACOLOGY
Shiitake mycelia is rich in carbohydrates, protein, vitamins and minerals. The polysaccharide-protein complex is a principle component of the extract, and provides significant immune support. Key therapeutic substances of shiitake mycelia are a new peptidomannan, KS-2, and a water solubilized linin derivative, EPS-3, which has antiviral activity, especially against herpes simplex types 1 and 2, and western equine encephalitis.

ACTIVE PROPERTIES
Shiitake mycelia or its alcohol precipitate fraction enhance immunity in the following ways:
1. activate macrophages, promoting recognition of antigens and information transmission to the helper T-cells, and increasing rate at which objects are engulfed;
2. reinforce interleukin-1 production, activating the helper T-cells;
3. promote the mitosis of B-lymphocytes (and others), increasing their proliferation;
4. increase antibody production.

PROCESSING
The high KS-2 extract is produced by liquid culture fermentation of Lentinus edodes mycelia, separation of the mycelia by centrifuge, hot water extraction at 90°C., alcohol precipitation of the water extract, centrifuge separation of the alcohol precipitate, and evaporation under vacuum. The high KS-2 extract is a 28:1 concentration; one gram of extract is equivalent to 28 grams of dried shiitake mycelia.

DIRECTIONS FOR USE
For general tonification and protection, 100 mg to 400 mg extract daily, between meals. Estimate for therapeutic use: 1.8 to 9 grams extract daily for several months, then taper back to 1/4 to 1/2 that amount daily, or as recommended by a health care practitioner. A successful study (especially, improved lymphocyte blastogenesis reaction) with HIV-infected hemophiliacs used 3 grams of LEM® (payented Lentinus edodes Mycelia extract), three times daily (total 9 grams).

HISTORICAL USES

- Cancer
- high cholesterol
- diseases of the liver such as hepatitis-B and cirrhosis
- general immune response support
- diabetes (for high cholesterol)
- HIV infection (for immune support)

SHIITAKE MYCELIA EXTRACT

TOXICITY, CAUTIONS & CONTRAINDICATIONS

No known toxicity. Tests on mice given up to 25 grams LEM per kilogram body weight by stomach tube produced no deaths, and only transient, mild depression of motor activity and soft feces (which would follow from the high fiber content).

SCIENTIFIC REFERENCES

• Sorimachi, K., et al., Anti-Viral Activity of Water-solubilized Lignin Derivatives in vitro, Agri. Biol. Chem., vol.54(5), pp.1337-1339, 1990.
• Mizoguchi, Y., et al., Determination of IL-1 Activity in the Supernatant of a Macrophage Culture Treated with LEM, Kantansui, vol. 15(1), pp. 127-135, 1987.
• Mizoguchi, Y., The Effects of LEM on the Induction of anti-TNP-SRBC Antibody Producing Cells by PWM Stimulation, Kantansui, vol. 15(1), pp. 127-135, 1987.
• Masayasu, N., et al., The Effects of the Alcohol Deposit Fraction LAP of LEM in Reinforcing the Macrophages Phagocytosis Ability, J. Japanese Reticuloendothelial System Res. Assoc., vol. 27(1), pp. 201-207, 1987.
• Sugano, N., et al., The Lymphocyte Rejuvenation Ability of the Polysaccharide Protein Fraction LAP-1 Obtained from a LEM Culture Base, Nihon Yakugakkai, 105th Annual Meeting.
• Suzuki, R., et al., Antiviral and interferon-producing activities of a new peptidomannan, KS-2, extracted from culture mycelia of lentinus edodes, J. of Antibiotics, vol.32, pg. 1336, 1979.
• Harada, T., & Kanetaka, T., [oral administration of LEM with EP3 improved the hepatic functions of hepatitis-B patients in vivo without serious side effects] Kantansui, vol.14, pg.327, 1987.
• Tochikura, T.S., et al., Inhibition (in vitro) of replication and of the cyptopathic effect of human immunodeficiency virus by an extract of the culture medium of Lentinus edodes mycelia, Med. Microbiol. Immunol., vol. 177, pp.235-244, 1988.
• Kanemoto, M., Acute Oral Toxicity Study of Lentinus Edodes Mycelial Powder (Moncelium rtm powder) in Male and Female Mice, Biotechnical Research Laboratories, Inc., Tech. Report No. 830916A, Oct. 20, 1983.

ANALYSIS

Potency–Polysaccharides, by column chromatography:	3.2% pure KS-2
Concentration	28:1 (28 g dried mycelia / 1 g extract)
Moisture	<5.0%
Protein	18.1%
Lipids	4.8%
Carbohydrates	47.1%
Ash	24.5%
Minerals (mg/gm)	
Phosphorus	75.2
Potassium	42.0
Magnesium	6.25
Heavy Metals (mcg /gm)	
Lead	8.5
Cadmium	none detected (nd)
Arsenic	nd
Mercury	nd
Microbiological Total Plate count	<=5,000cfu/gm
Total Coliform	neg
Pesticides	neg. for organochlorines

ST. JOHN'S WORT

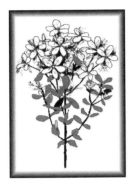

DESCRIPTION

St. John's wort is a perennial with regular flowers which bloom from June until September. The plant was believed, from the time of the ancient Greeks until the Middle Ages, to ward off witchcraft and evil spirits and to drive out devils. Considered a noxious weed by farmers due to its photosensitizing effect on livestock, St. John's wort has nevertheless been used by humans for centuries for a wide variety of ailments, including nervous disorders, depression, neuralgia, wounds and burns, kidney problems, and for its anti-bacterial and anti-inflammatory actions. Recently a great deal of attention has been placed on the herb because of its two main active ingredients, hypericin and pseudohypericin, which have been shown to inhibit the AIDS virus.

PHARMACOLOGY

St. John's wort contains a variety of active ingredients including dianthrone derivatives (hypericin and pseudohypericin), flavonoids and tannins (hyperoside, quercetin, rutin, catechin), xanthrones, monoterpenes and sesquiterpenes, and phytosterols (beta-sitosterol). Xanthrones and hypericin have been shown to have monoamine-oxidase (MAO)-inhibiting activity. A standard treatment for depression uses MAO inhibitors to retard the breakdown of neurotransmitters such as norepinephrine and serotonin and thus increase their concentration in the central nervous system. A clinical trial involving standardized hypericin extract showed improvement in depressive symptoms, including anxiety, apathy, insomnia, depression, and feelings of worthlessness. The flavonoids and possibly other agents have wound healing and anti-inflammatory activities. Most current research has focused on the antiviral activity of the anthroquinones, hypericin and pseudohypericin. Hypericin is a photodynamic red pigment whose anti-viral activity is substantially enhanced by exposure to light. The mechanism is thought to involve the production of oxygen free-redicals which can damage the vi-

COMMON NAME
St. John's Wort, Goatweed
Hypericum, Klamath weed
LATIN NAME
Hypericum perforatum
ORIGIN
Worldwide
PART OF PLANT USED
Aerial parts
ACTIVE SUBSTANCES
Glycosides (hypericin, pseudohypericin), flavonoids, tannins
STANDARD
0.3%-0.5% Hypericin

HISTORICAL USES

- Depression, psychological illness, mania, fear, nervous disorders, hysteria
- Sedative
- Wound and burn healing (external)
- Anti-bacterial
- Anti-viral, AIDS
- Bed-wetting, childhood nightmares
- Gastritis, gastric ulcers, inflammatory bowel disorders
- Inflammation
- Myalgias (external)
- Neuralgia, sciatica (external)
- Kidney, genito-urinary troubles
- Diuretic
- Menstrual cramps

ST. JOHN'S WORT

ral envelope. Non-enveloped viruses such as polio or adenovirus are unaffected by hypericin. The human studies involved taking high doses of hypericin (10 mg) extracted from St. John's wort.

ACTIVE PROPERTIES

St. John's wort has been used for centuries to calm the nerves and treat depression. A vivid red oil made from macerating the flowers in vegetable oil has been used to dress wounds, heal deep cuts, soothe burns and ease the pain of neuralgias. Taken internally, the oil has been used for ulcers and gastritis. An infusion of the herb has also been used as an expectorant for bronchitis and as a diuretic for the kidneys and as an easing agent for menstrual cramps.

DIRECTIONS FOR USE

250 mg. extract / day

BIO-ENHANCING AGENTS

Beta-carotene, vitamin C

TOXICITY, CAUTIONS & CONTRA-INDICATIONS

Consumption of hypericin may render the skin photosensitive. Care should be taken during exposure to sunlight. Avoid excessive exposure to sunlight, tanning lights or UV sources.

PROCESSING

The aerial portions of St. John's wort are harvested, dried away from sunlight and extracted with ethanol and water.

SCIENTIFIC REFERENCES

• Gerhardt, J.J. and Fowkes, S.W. (1991) Hypericin. J. Theor. and Applied Health Techn. 6(6), #31:1.
• Hobbs, C. (1989) St. John's wort. A reveiew. HerbalGram 18/19:24.
• Lopez-Bazzocchi, I. et al. (1991) Antiviral activity of the photoactive plant pigment hypericin. Photochem. and Photobiol. 54(1):95.
• Meruelo, D. et al. (1988) Therapeutic agents with dramatic anti-retroviral activity and little toxicity at effective doses: Aromatic polycyclic diones hypericin and pseudohypericin. Proc. Natl. Acad. Sci.(USA) 85:5230
• Muldner, Von H. and Zoller, M. (1984) Antidepressive activity of an hypericin standardized extract of Hypericum. Arzneim. Forschh./Drug. Res. 34:918.
• Schinazi, R.F. et al. (1990) Anthaquinones as a new class of antiviral agents against human immunodeficiency virus. Antivial Res. 13:265.
• Suzuki, O. et al. (1984) Inhibition of monoamine oxidase by hypericin. Planta medica 50:272.
• Weiner, M. (1990) Weiner's Herbal. Mill Valley: Quantum Books.

ANALYSIS

Product	St. John's wort
Type	Standardized extract
Standardization	53-58 mg /100 g Hypericine
Character	dark brown-red fine powder
Loss on drying	max. 5.0
Solubility	cloudy water soluble
Heavy Metals	< 62 ppm

SUMA
(Pffafia Paniculata)

COMMON NAME
Brazilian Ginseng, Para Todo
LATIN NAME
Pffafia paniculata
FAMILY
Amaranthaceae
ORIGIN
Brazil
PART OF PLANT USED
Roots
ACTIVE SUBSTANCES
Saponins: Pffafosides A,B,C,
D,E,F and Pffafic Acid
STANDARD
5% Beta Ecdysone

DESCRIPTION
Suma is one of the most highly regarded herbs from South America and is native to the mid-Atlantic Forest region of the Sao Paulo and Rio de Janiero states. The plant consists of a ground covering vine with an intricate and deep root structure. Suma is considered to be a true adaptogen and has been used by native peoples for centuries. In the past two decades a great deal has been learned about the phytochemistry and pharmacology of this plant and its constituents.

PHARMACOLOGY
Suma is used mostly as an adaptogen. Adaptogens exert a normalizing influence on the body, increasing resistance to stress. Studies have shown anabolic, analgesic and anti-inflammatory effects. It is a tonic and a nutrient and has been traditionally used topically for regenerative effects.

ACTIVE PROPERTIES
Among the many ingredients found in Suma, the most notable is Ecdysterone. Also known as B-ecdysterone, this phytosterol or plant hormone is very similiar in use to alpha-ecdysone, an insect molting hormone. Suma is considered to be one of the richest sources of B-ecdysterone. Ecdysones and plant sterols in general, have been the focus of a great deal of research all over the world for their anabolic effects and a variety of applications. Other phytosterols found in Suma include Beta-Sitosterol, Polypodine b and Stigmasterol. There are many other nutrients found in this plant, including a broad spectrum of vitamins, minerals and amino acids. Allantoin, a cell building compound, and trace amounts of germanium are also found. Other active constiuents include six unique saponins called pfaffosides (pfaffosides A-F), as well as pfaffic acid. As much as 30% (by weight) of the whole root consists of dietary fiber.

DIRECTIONS FOR USE
1-2 200 mg. capsules per day

TOXICITY, CAUTIONS & CONTRA-INDICATIONS
Suma shows very low toxicity and does not appear to cause adverse reactions. Beta-ecdysone has an LD50 of 9gr/kg for oral ingestion in mice. Because of Suma's natural hormones it should not be taken during pregnancy.

HISTORICAL USES

- Anabolic
- Analgesic
- Anti-inflammatory
- Tonic and nutrient for regeneration
- Increases resistance to stress

SUMA

PROCESSING

This product is prepared by distilling and spraying an extract of Suma using a 96% pure sugar cane ethanol. The resulting powder has a minimum of 5% Beta-ecdysone.

SCIENTIFIC REFERENCES

• RTECS (number FZ80600)
• Hikino, H. and Takemoto, T., Naturwissenschaften, 59:91-98 1972
• Otaka, T. and others, Chem. Pharm. Bull., 17:1352-1355.
• Syrov, V.V. Med. Zh. Uzb., 3:67-9 1986
• Kurmukov, A.G., Med. Zh. Uzb. ISS 10 68-70 1988

ANALYSIS

Product	Suma
Type	Standardized extract
Standardization	5% Beta-ecdysone
Character	dry tan powder
Taste	characteristic
Germanium	traces
Vitamins	A, E, B-1, B-2
Saponins	Pfaffosides A-F and Pfaffic Acid
Heavy Metals	< 20 ppm
Microbiological Specifications	
gram negatives	absent
E. coli	absent
staph aureus	absent
psedomonas aeruginosa	absent
salmonella	absent

TURMERIC

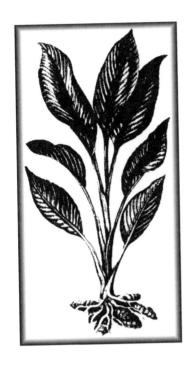

COMMON NAME
Turmeric
LATIN NAME
Curcuma longa
ORIGIN
India
PART OF PLANT USED
Rhizome
ACTIVE SUBSTANCES
curcumin, essential oil
(p-tolymethylcarbinol)
STANDARD
95% curcumin

DESCRIPTION

Turmeric has long been considered an essential flavoring spice of Indian and other ethnic cuisines. Turmeric provides the typical yellow color of many curry dishes and helps to render food more digestible. Turmeric along with other curry herbs has several physiologic activities, including the inhibition of platelet aggregation, antibiotic effects, anti-cholesterol action and fibrinolytic activity.

PHARMACOLOGY

Many studies on Turmeric have revealed that the herb contains cholagogue-type substances which increase the secretion of bile. Principal among these substances is curcumin. Curcumin also possesses liver protective activity, detoxifying dangerous carcinogens, stimulating the gall bladder, and acting as a free-radical scavenger. Curcumin has cholekinetic activity (bile duct stimulation). It has been suggested that Turmeric lowers blood cholesterol through these various choleretic effects. Turmeric's effects on weight loss may also be mediated through curcumin's catabolic and metabolic activities on fats. Studies have also revealed that curcumin has anti-inflammatory properties, inhibiting platelet aggregation and cyclooxgenase and lipoxygenase enzymes which catalyze the formation of inflammatory prostaglandins and molecules. Curcumin requires the presence of the adrenal glands to have this non-steroidal anti-inflammatory activity.

ACTIVE PROPERTIES

Turmeric has long been used in folk medicine to treat arthritis, lower blood cholesterol, stimulate digestion, protect the liver, and treat obesity. Turmeric also has strong antibacterial and antifungal properties.

DIRECTIONS FOR USE

100 mg. / with meals.

BIO-ENHANCING AGENTS

Dandelion root, milk thistle extract, licorice, artichoke, flavonoids.

TOXICITY, CAUTIONS & CONTRA-INDICATIONS

No known toxicity. Large doses are not recommended in cases of painful gall stones, obstructive jaundice, acute bilious colic and extremely toxic liver disorders.

HISTORICAL USES

- Hepatitis
- Indigestion
- Gallbladder or liver disease
- Bile duct problems
- Obesity
- Arthritis
- As a cholagogue
- As an anti-inflammatory
- Hepatoprotective
- As a gallbladder tonic
- As a cancer preventative

TURMERIC

SCIENTIFIC REFERENCES

• Azuine, M. et al. (1992) Protective role of aqueous turmeric extract against mutagenicity of direct-acting carcinogens as well as Benzo[a]pyrene-induced genotoxicity and carcinogenicity. J. Canc. Res. Clin. Oncol. 118:447-452.

• Charles, V. and Charles, S. (1992) The use and efficacy of Azadirachta indica ADR (NEEM) and curcuma longa (Turmeric) in scabies. Trop. and Geog. Med. 44:178.

• Mowrey, D. (1990) Guaranteed Potency Herbs. A compilation of writings on the subject.

• Soni, K. et al. (1992) Reversal of aflatoxin induced liver damage by turmeric and curcumin. Cancer Letters 115-121.

• Tonnesen, H.H. (1989) Studies on curcumin and curcuminoids. XIII. Catalytic effect of curcumin on the peroxidation of linoleic acid by 15-lipoxygenase. Int. J. Pharm. 50:67-69.

• Weiner, M. (1990) Weiner's Herbal, Mill Valley: Quantum Books.

ANALYSIS

Product	Turmeric
Type	Standardized extract
Standardization	95% curcumin
Character	bright yellow powder
Ash	4.9%
pH (c=5, water)	6.4
Heavy Metals	undetected
Microbiological Content	absent

UVA URSI

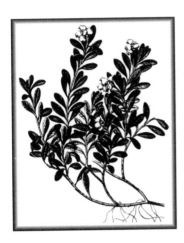

COMMON NAME
Uva ursi, Bearberry, Whortleberry, Bear's Grape, Kinnikinnick, Mountain cranberry, Mealberry

LATIN NAME
Arctostaphylos uva-ursi

ORIGIN
Northern United States and Europe

PART OF PLANT USED
Leaves

ACTIVE SUBSTANCES
Glycosides (Arbutin and methylarbutin), tannin, hydroquinone, allantoin

STANDARD
10% -25% Arbutin

DESCRIPTION
Uva ursi is a small perennial evergreen shrub. White flowers tinged with red blossom from June to September followed by small edible red berries. Uva ursi leaf is widely used as a diuretic, astringent, and antiseptic. Folk medicine around the world has recommended uva ursi for nephritis, kidney stones, and chronic cystitis. The herb has also been used as a general tonic for weakened kidneys, liver or pancreas.

PHARMACOLOGY
Uva ursi contains a high concentration of arbutin, an antiseptic phenolic glycoside. Arbutin and other glycosides have diuretic and urinary antiseptic action. They relieve pain from bladder stones, cystitis, nephritis, and kidney stones. Arbutin is converted in the body to hydroquinones and glucose which have antiseptic and disinfecting properties if the urine is alkaline. The hydroquinone will turn the urine green. Uva ursi also contains allantoin which is known for its soothing and tissue-repairing properties.

PROCESSING
The green leaves are picked in autumn and dried.

DIRECTIONS FOR USE
100-200 mg / day standardized extract

BIO-ENHANCING AGENTS
Cubeb, buchu, cowberry (vaccinium vitisisdea), rupturewort (herniaria glabra).

TOXICITY, CAUTIONS & CONTRA-INDICATIONS
Non toxic beyond the following cautions: Uva ursi requires an alkaline pH to work. It is contraindicated as a urinary disinfectant under conditions of acid urine. Urine can be made alkaline by ingesting a heaping teaspoon of bicarbonate of soda. Contra-indicated as a diuretic or flushing agent in acute cystitis. Can induce gastric irritation if overused due to the tannin concentration. Should not be used during pregnancy. Consumption of Uva-Ursi will turn the urine a harmless temporary green color.

HISTORICAL USES

- Cystitis, Nephritis, Pyelo-nephritis
- Catarrhal conditions in the urinary tract
- As a diuretic
- Kidney and bladder stones
- As a liver, kidney and pancreas tonic
- As an astringent
- As an antiseptic
- As an anti-scorbutic
- Profuse menstruation
- Chronic diarrhea

UVA URSI

SCIENTIFIC REFERENCES
• Benigni, R. (1948) The presence of antibiotic substances in the higher plants. Fitoterapia, 19(3):1-2.
• Mowrey, D. (1986) Guaranteed Potency Herbs. A compilation of writings on the subject.
• Mowrey, D. (1986) The Scientific Validation of Herbal Medicine. Cormorant Books.
• Weiner, M. (1990) Weiner's Herbal. Mill Valley: Quantum Books.

ANALYSIS

Product	Uva Ursi
Type	Standardized extract
Standardization	25% arbutin
Character	brownflowable powder
Loss on drying	1.0%
Ash	2.4%
Solubility in water	98.9%
Heavy metals:	
Lead	<.28 mg/kg
Cadmium	<0.02 mg/kg
Mercury	<0.006 mg/kg
Aerobic plate count	none cfu /g
E. coli	absent
salmonella	absent
staph aureas	absent

VALERIAN

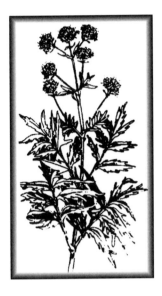

DESCRIPTION
Since ancient Greek times, valerian root has been valued as an antispasmodic and sleep aid. The first known records reported its use in the treatment of epilepsy. Today, valerian is widely used throughout Europe as a mild sedative and sleep aid for insomnia, and as a balancing agent for hyperexcitability and exhaustion, calming the one and stimulating the other.

PHARMACOLOGY
The sedative effects of Valerian root are attributed to the valepotriates, a group of unstable esters whose degradation products also possess sedative activity. Other components, particularly those of the pungent essential oil, the valerenic and isovaleric acids have sedative effects and central nervous system (CNS) depressant activity. Researchers have also established that the valepotriates and the other components of valerian possess relaxing and spasmolytic effects on smooth muscle. A mechanism has been proposed for the central nervous system effects involving the metabolism of gamma-aminobutyric acid (GABA) in the brain. Valerian appears the most effective when all its constituents are present. The different activities of valerian appear to be due to a complex mixture of substances.

ACTIVE PROPERTIES
Numerous clinical trials have been performed with valerian root and have found both subjective and objective improvements in emotional tension disturbances, sleep quality, and behavioral disorders without producing a hangover type effect the next morning.

PROCESSING
The root is collected in spring or autumn and dried. Cold percolation with ethanol / water. Evaporation at low temperature.

DIRECTIONS FOR USE
2.5 gm of root / day; 200 mg. extract, 1 tsp. tincture, repeated several times if needed.

COMMON NAME
Valerian Root
LATIN NAME
Valeriana officinalis
ORIGIN
Europe
PART OF PLANT USED
Rhizome, Root-stock
ACTIVE SUBSTANCES
Valepotriates, valeric acid, sesquiterpenes, glycoside, essential oils
STANDARD
.8%-1% Valeric acid
or valerenic acid

HISTORICAL USES

- Insomnia, especially due to nervous exhaustion
- Motoric restlessness or vegetative dysfunction
- Headaches
- Anxiety
- Nervous tension
- Palpitations
- High blood pressure
- As an antispasmodic
- Nervous dyspepsia, stomach cramps
- Spastic or irritable bowel
- Menstrual cramps
- Dandruff
- Epilepsy
- Childhood behavior disorders and learning disabilities

VALERIAN

BIO-ENHANCING AGENTS
Passion Flower, Hops, Chamomile, Hawthorn Berries

TOXICITY, CAUTIONS & CONTRA-INDICATIONS
No known toxicity. High doses (5 gms. root / day) can lead to minor withdrawal symptoms if taken over a long period of time. Avoid large doses and prolonged use.

SCIENTIFIC REFERENCES
• Boeters, U. (1969) Treatment of autonomic dysregulation with valepotriates (Valmane). Muenchener Medizinische Wochenschrift. 37:1873.
• Chauffard, F. et al. (1982) Detection of mild sedative effects: Valerian and sleep in man. Experimentia 37:622.
• Delsignore, R. et al. (1980) Placebo controlled clinical trial with Valerian. Settimana Medica 68(9):437.
• Drieglsten, J. and Grusla, D. (1988) Central depressant constituent in Valerian. Deutsche Apotheker Zeitung. 40:2041.
• Foster, S. (1991) Valerian. American Botanical Council.
• Hendriks, R. et al. (1981) Pharmacological screening of Valerenal and some other components of essential oil of *Valeriana officinalis*. Planta Medica 42:62.
• Klich, R. and Gladbach, B. (1975) Childhood behavior disorders and their treatment. Medizinische Welt. 26(25):1251.
• Lindahl, O. and Lindwall, L. (1989) Double blind study of a valerian preparation. Pharmacology Biochem. & Behavior. 32:1065.
• Mowrey, D. (1990) Guaranteed Potency Herbs. A compilation of writings on the subject.
• Mowrey, D. (1986) The Scientific Validation of Herbal Medicine. Cormorant Books.
• Weiner, M. (1990) Weiner's Herbal. Mill Valley: Quantum Books.

ANALYSIS

Product	Valerian Root
Type	Standardized extract
Standardization	.92% valerenic acid
Character	brown powder
Ash	5.24%
Water (K.Fischer)	2.53%
Heavy Metals	<100.0 ppm
Microbiological Content	<1000. cfu/g
Fungi	<100.0 cfu/g
Staph. aureas	absent
E. coli	absent
salmonella	absent

WILLOW BARK

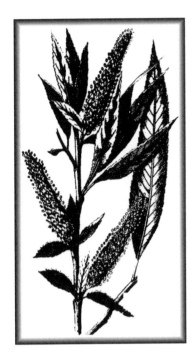

COMMON NAME
White Willow, Pussy Willow, Purple Willow

LATIN NAME
Salax alba, Salix purpurea L.

ORIGIN
Europe, Yugoslavia

PART OF PLANT USED
Bark (cortex)

ACTIVE SUBSTANCES
phenolic glycosides, (salicin, salicortin, tremulacin, fragilin, salicoylsalicin, salireposide), tannins, syringin, flavonoid glycosides (isorhamnetin, quercetin)

STANDARD
8% Salicin

DESCRIPTION
The bark of the common Willow tree has been known since antiquity for its pain-relieving and fever-reducing properties. In the early 19th century a French chemist extracted the principal active ingredient from Willow Bark and named it Salicin. At the end of the century, Felix Hofmann, a chemist at the Bayer company in Germany developed the world's most used medication, aspirin or acetyl-salicylic acid. Recently, however, pain sufferers are returning to the natural source to avoid the potentially dangerous side effects of aspirin.

PHARMACOLOGY
Willow Bark contains bitter phenolic and flavonoid glycosides. The most famous and active phenolic glycoside is salicin, which is a monoglycoside of salicylic acid. Salicylic acid is a weak anti-inflammatory agent but is converted by the liver to acetyl-salicylic acid. The acetylated version has aspirin's more effective anti-inflammatory activity without its gastrointestinal toxicity. The salicylates inhibit the activity of the cyclo-oxgenase enzyme and thus inhibit the production of prostaglandins and other inflammatory molecules.

ACTIVE PROPERTIES
Willow bark has long been used for fevers and inflammations. In addition, the astringency of the glycosides makes willow bark useful as an antiseptic and astringent. Extracts and infusions of the bark have been used for cleansing the scalp and skin, for treating dandruff, and for treating corns and growths.

PROCESSING
The bark is peeled from the trees without damaging them and dried, then extracted with 80% ethanol and 20% water, followed by a pH adjustment and evaporation at room temperature at reduced pressure.

DIRECTIONS FOR USE
60-120 mg. salicin
750-1500 mg. / day extract

BIO-ENHANCING AGENTS
Rosemary Leaf, Skullcap, Blue Vervain.

TOXICITY, CAUTIONS & CONTRA-INDICATIONS
None known. Individuals allergic to salicylates should avoid willow bark.

HISTORICAL USES

- Temporary use in pain: headache, menstrual pain, toothache, arthritis, gout, angina, sore muscles
- Antiseptic for urinary tract infections
- Fevers, rheumatic conditions
- Inflammatory pain
- Connective tissue disorders
- As an astringent for dysentery, diarrhea, intestinal worms and parasites

WILLOW BARK

SCIENTIFIC REFERENCES
• Julkunen-Tiito, R. and Tahvanainen, J. (1989) The effect of sample preparation method of extractable phenolics of Salicaceae species. Planta Medica 55:55.
• Mowrey, D. (1986) The Scientific Validation of Herbal Medicine. Cormorant Books.
• Vane, J.R. (1971) Salicylates. Nature 231:232.
• Weiner, M. (1990) Weiner's Herbal. Mill Valley: Quantum Books.

ANALYSIS

Product	Willow Bark Extract
Type	Standardized extract
Standardization	7.8% Salicin (HPLC)
Drug/Extract Ratio	6,4-8,0-1
Plant Material	Cortex
Character	yellow-brown fine powder
Content	Salicine: 8.1% (HPLC)
Loss on drying	4.2% m/m
Bulk Density	0.44 g/ml
Preserving Agent	none
Microbiological Content	
Aerobic microorg.	180n / g
molds/yeasts <100/g	complies
enterobacteria <100/g	complies
Salmonella n.n/50g	complies
Pseudomonas aer. n.n/g	complies
E. coli n.n/g	complies
Staphylococcus a. n.n/g	complies
Pestiside residues	accord. to Purity Data Sheet

INDEX

Blood Sugar (Low)	DGL (Licorice)
Blood Sugar Regulation	American Ginseng, Siberian Ginseng
Boils	Echinacea
Bone-Flesh-Cartilage	Gotu Kola, Willow Bark (pain)
Bronchitis	Chinese Garlic, Goldenseal, Licorice, Saw Palmetto
Bronchodilator	Ephedra (Ma Huang)
Burn Healing	St. John's Wort

C

Calming agent	Chamomile
Cancer preventative	Reishi Mushroom Extract, Turmeric
Candida	Goldenseal (douche)
Capillary fragility	Bilberry, Green Tea Extract
Cataracts	Bilberry
Catarrhal conditions	Goldenseal, Saw Palmetto
Cathartic	Cascara Sagrada
Cavities	Green Tea Extract
Cellulite	Gotu Kola
Cellulitis	Gotu Kola
Cerebral vascular insuffic.	Ginkgo Biloba, Grape Seed Extract
Chapped skin	Chamomile (external)
Chills	Ephedra (Ma Huang)
Cholalogue	Cascara Sagrada, Milk Thistle, Turmeric
Cholesterol Regulation	Artichoke, Milk Thistle, Turmeric
Cholesterol (high) Shiitake Mycelia	Chinese Garlic, Ginger, Korean Ginseng, Green Tea Extarct,Dong Quai, Reishi Mushroom,
Chronic Fatigue Syndrome	Reishi Mushroom Extract
Circulation	Astragalus, Bilberry, Butcher's Broom, Chinese Garlic, Ephedra (Ma Huang), Ginkgo Biloba, Gotu Kola, Hawthorne, Korean Ginseng,
Cirrhosis	Licorice, Shiitake Mycelia Extract,
Climacteric Disoders	Hops
CNS depressant	American Ginseng
CNS stimulant	Guarana, Kola Nut (caffeine), Korean Ginseng
CNS vascular disturbances	Bilberry
Colds	Chinese Garlic, Echinacea, Saw Palmetto
Concentration	Passion Flower, Schisandra, Siberian Ginseng
Confinement	Gotu Kola
Connective Tissue Disorders	Willow Bark (pain)
Constipation	Licorice
Convalescence	American Ginseng, Dong Quai (women), Nettles, Shiitake Mycelia, Siberian Ginseng
Cortisol Release	Echinacea
Cough	Ephedra (Ma Huang)(in Feverish states), Licorice
Crohn's Disease	Hops
Cystitis	Horsetail, Uva Ursi
Cuts	Chamomile (external), Chinese Garlic

D

Dandruff	Valerian
Debility	American Ginseng, Dong Quai, Horsetail, Nettles, Siberian Ginseng
Dementia	Ginkgo Biloba
Depression	Feverfew, Schisandra, Siberian Ginseng, St. John's Wort
Dermatitis	Chamomile (external), Licorice
Detoxify/Nurture	Echinacea
Diabetes	Bilberry, Butcher's Broom, Ginkgo Biloba, Gotu Kola, Grape Seed Extract, Shiitake Mycelia,
Diabetic-induced cataracts	Bilberry
Diabetic retinopathy	Butcher's Broom
Diaphoretic	Chamomile
Diarrhea	Goldenseal, Guarana, Hawthorne, Uva Ursi, Willow Bark,
Digestion	American Ginseng,Artichoke, Chinese Garlic, Devil's Claw, Feverfew, Ginger, Goldenseal, Green Tea Extract, Guarana, Hawthorne, Hops, Licorice, Milk Thistle, Reishi Mushroom Extract, Saw Palmetto, Schisandra,Turmeric
Diuretic	Artichoke, Ephedra (Ma Huang), Hops, Horsetail, Nettles, St. John's Wort
Diverticulitis	Chamomile

Dizziness	Ginkgo Biloba, Schisandra
Dry skin	Chamomile (external)
Dysentery	Chinese Garlic, Willow Bark
Dysmenorrhea (cramps)	Agnus Castus, Dong Quai, St. John's Wort
Dyspepsia	Devil's Claw, Ginger, Goldenseal, Hawthorne, Valerian
Dysuria	Pygeum

E

Ear infections	Echinacea
Eczema	Chamomile (external), Goldenseal, Nettles
Edema	Devil's Claw, Dong Quai, Echinacea, Ginkgo Biloba, Gotu Kola, Grape Seed Extract
Emmenagogue	Feverfew
Endometriosis	Agnus Castus
Endurance	Schisandra
Enuresis	Ephedra (Ma Huang), Saw Palmetto
Environmental Pollution	Ginseng
Epilepsy	Valerian
Episiotomy tears	Gotu Kola
Erectile dysfunction	Ginkgo Biloba
Erysepilas	Gotu Kola
Exhaustion	Korean Ginseng, Nettles, Valerian
Expectorant	Chinese Garlic, Saw Palmetto
Eyes	Bilberry, Schisandra
Eye infections	Echinacea, Goldenseal

F

Fatigue	American Ginseng, Ginkgo Biloba, Gotu Kola, Guarana, Kola Nut, Korean Ginseng, Reishi Mushroom Extract, Siberian Ginseng
Fear, excessive	St. John's Wort
Female Tonic	American Ginseng, Gotu Kola, Licorice
Fertility	Siberian Ginseng
Fertility (male)	Korean Ginseng
Fever (acute)	American Ginseng, Feverfew, Willow Bark
Flatulence	Chamomile, Ginger, Goldenseal
Food Poisoning	Green Tea Extract
Flu	Chinese Garlic, Echinacea

G

Gall Bladder problems	Devil's Claw, Goldenseal, Milk Thistle, Turmeric
Gangrene	Echinacea
Gastritis	Chamomile, Chinese Garlic, Goldenseal, St. John's Wort
Gastrointestinal problems	American Ginseng, Goldenseal, St. John's Wort
Gingivitis	Chamomile (external)
Gonorrhea	Goldenseal
Gout	Devil's Claw, Nettles, Willow Bark (pain)
Gums	Bilberry, Echinacea

H

Hair (lifeless, loss)	Horsetail, Nettles
Hayfever & Allergy	Echinacea, Siberian Ginseng, Nettles
Headaches (tension)	Feverfew, Ginkgo Biloba, Guarana, Kava Kava, Valerian, Willow Bark
Heart Tonic	Bilberry, Butcher's Broom, Ginkgo Biloba, Gotu Kola, Hawthorne, Korean Ginseng
Heartbeats (irregular)	Hawthorne
Heartburn	Chamomile, Goldenseal

Hemorrhages	Bilberry, Butcher's Broom, Goldenseal
Hemorrhoids	Bilberry, Butcher's Broom, Ginkgo Biloba, Gotu Kola, Passion Flower
Hepatitis (acute, chronic)	Milk Thistle, Shiitake Mycelia Extract, Turmeric
Hepatoprotective	Milk Thistle, Shiitake Mycelia Extarct, Turmeric
High Altitude Sickness	Ginkgo Biloba, Reishi Mushroom Extract
High Blood Pressure	Dong Quai, Green Tea Extract, Reishi Mushroom Extract
High Cholesterol	Dong Quai, Green Tea Extract, Shiitake Mycelia Extract
HIV (immune support)	Shiitake Mycelia Extract
Hyperactivity	Passion Flower, Valerian
Hyperglycemia	Siberian Ginseng
Hypertension	American Ginseng, Astragalus, Bilberry, Hawthorne
Hypoglycemia	Licorice, Siberian Ginseng
Hypotension	Ephedra (Ma Huang)
Hypoxia, Altitude Sickness	Ginkgo Biloba, Schisandra
Hysteria	St. John's Wort

I

Immune system	Astragalus, Devil's Claw, Dong Quai, Echinacea, Horsetail, Korean Ginseng, Reishi Mushroom Extract, Siberian Ginseng, Shiitake Mycelia Extract,
Immunostimulatory	American Ginseng, Devil's Claw, Dong Quai, Echinacea, Horsetail, Korean Ginseng, Siberian Ginseng,
Impetigo	Goldenseal, Licorice
Impotence	Ginkgo Biloba, Saw Palmetto
Incontinence	Pygeum
Indigestion	Devil's Claw, Ginger, Hawthorne, Hops, Reishi Mushroom Extract, Turmeric
Infections Siberian Ginseng	Astragalus, Chamomile, Chinese Garlic, Echinacea, Goldenseal, Gotu Kola, Licorice,
Infertility	American Ginseng, Saw Palmetto (women)
Inflammation	American Ginseng, Chamomile, Dong Quai, Echinacea, Feverfew, Ginkgo Biloba, Goldenseal, Hops, DGL (Licorice), Nettles, Passion Flower, St. John's Wort, Willow Bark
Inflammatory Bowel Disorders	St. John's Wort
Influenza	Echinacea
Insect bites	Echinacea
Insomnia	American Ginseng, Chamomile, Feverfew, Hawthorne, Hops, Passion Flower, Reishi Mushroom Extract, Schisandra, Valerian
Intermittent Claudication	Dong Quai
Irritable Bowel Syndrome	Hops, Valerian
Ischemia	Ginkgo Biloba

J

Jaundice	Milk Thistle

K

Kidney	Artichoke, Devil's Claw, Milk Thistle, St. John's Wort, Schisandra, Uva Ursi
Kidney Hematuria	Bilberry
Kidney stones	Schisandra, Uva Ursi

L

Lactation	Hops, Nettles, Saw Palmetto
Laxative	Cascara Sagrada, Licorice, Milk Thistle
Learning	Gotu Kola
Libido (low)	Saw Palmetto, Schisandra
Liver Disorders, liver tonics	Artichoke, Cascara Sagrada, Chinese Garlic, Devil's Claw, Dong Quai, Feverfew, Goldenseal, Licorice, Milk Thistle, Schisandra, Turmeric,
Liver, fatty degeneration	Milk Thistle
Lumbago	Nettles
Lung complaints	Horsetail, Reishi Mushroom Extract, Schisandra

M

Mania	St. John's Wort
Memory	Ginkgo Biloba, Gotu Kola, Schisandra
Menopause	Agnus Castus, Dong Quai, Passion Flower
Menstrual problems	Agnus Castus, Butcher's Broom, Dong Quai, Feverfew, Goldenseal, Milk Thistle, Nettles,

	Passion Flower, Saw Palmetto, Uva Ursi
Menstrual cramps	Chamomile, Dong Quai, Saw Palmetto, St. John's Wort, Valerian, Willow Bark
Mental Alertness/Senility	Gingko Biloba, Gotu Kola, Korean Ginseng, Passion Flower, Schisandra, Siberian Ginseng
Migraines	Feverfew, Ginkgo Biloba
Morning Sickness	Ginger
Motion Sickness	Ginger
Muscles (sore)	Willow Bark
Myalgias	St. John's Wort, Willow Bark
Myasthenia gravis	Astragalus
Myopia	Bilberry

N

Nails	Horsetail
Nasal congestion	Ephedra (Ma Huang)
Nausea	Feverfew, Ginger, Turmeric
Near-sightedness	Schisandra
Nephritis	Uva Ursi
Nervous Breakdown	Siberian Ginseng, St. John's Wort
Nervous Tension	American Ginseng, Chamomile, Gingko Biloba, Guarana, Hawthorne, Hops, Korean Ginseng, Passion Flower, Siberian Ginseng, St. John's Wort, Valerian
Neuralgia	Guarana, St. John's Wort,
Neurasthenia	Schisandra
Night Vision	Bilberry
Nightmares	St. John's Wort
Nocturnal cramps	Gotu Kola
Numbness	Ginkgo Biloba
Nycturia	Pygeum, Saw Palmetto

O

Obesity	Turmeric
Ovarian Function	Saw Palmetto

P

Pain Relief (temporary)	Devil's Claw, Dong Quai, Echinacea, Guarana, Willow Bark
Palpitations	Schisandra, Valerian
Pancreatic tonic	Uva Ursi
Paradentosis	Chamomile (external)
Parasites	Chinese Garlic, Goldenseal, Willow Bark
Parturition	Passion Flower
Perineal lesions/delivery	Gotu Kola
Peripheral Arterial Insufficiency	Ginkgo Biloba
Peripheral Vascular Disease	Astragalus, Dong Quai, Ginkgo Biloba
Pharyngitis	Chamomile (external)
Phlebitis	Bilberry, Gotu Kola
Physical performance	Korean Ginseng, Siberian Ginseng
Pigmentary retinitis	Bilberry
PMS	Agnus Castus, Dong Quai
Pneumonia	Chinese Garlic
Pollution	Siberian Ginseng
Polynephritis	Uva Ursi
Polyuria	Pygeum
Post-thrombotic syndrome	Butcher's Broom
Pregnancy cramps	Butcher's Broom
Pregnancy lesions	Gotu Kola)
Proctitis	Butcher's Broom
Proctology	Butcher's Broom
Prostate Cancer	Pygeum
Prostate Problems	Horsetail, Korean Ginseng, Nettles, Pygeum, Saw Palmetto, Turmeric
Proteinuria	Artichoke
Pruritis ani (anal itching)	Butcher's Broom
Psoriasis	Milk Thistle
Psychosis	American Ginseng, St. John's Wort
Pulmonary Tuberculosis	Horsetail

Purgative	Cascara Sagrada

R

Radioprotective	Korean Ginseng, Reishi Mushroom Extract
Rashes	Licorice
Raynaud's syndrome	Ginkgo Biloba, Hawthorne
Relaxation	American Ginseng, Chamomile, Kava Kava
Rectal Inflammations	Goldenseal
Respiratory Ailments	Echinacea, Ephedra (Ma Huang), Green Tea Extract
Restlessness	Chamomile, Feverfew, Hops, Valerian
Restorative	Korean Ginseng, Suma
Retinal Disturbances	Bilberry, Butcher's Broom, Grape Seed Extract
Rheumatism	Devil's Claw, Willow Bark
Rhinitis	Goldenseal, Nettles
Ringworm	Goldenseal

S

Sciatica	Nettles, St. John's Wort
Sedative	American Ginseng, Chamomile, Devil's Claw, Dong Quai , Echinacea, Feverfew, Goldenseal, Gotu Kola, Hops, Kava Kava, Passion Flower, St. John's Wort, Saw Palmetto
Shampoo	Horsetail
Sinus Congestion	Nettles
Sinusitis	Nettles
Skin, chapped	Chamomile (external)
Skin Disorders	Bilberry, Butcher's Broom, Gotu Kola, Echinacea, Horsetail, Licorice
Skin Infections	Goldenseal, Gotu Kola, Licorice
Skin Injuries	Gotu Kola
Snake Bites	Echinacea
Sores	Chamomile (external), Echinacea, Gotu Kola
Sore Throats	Echinacea
Spastic Colon	Valerian
Spleen tonic	Milk Thistle
Spondylosis-/lower back pain	Devil's Claw
Sterility	Siberian Ginseng
Stimulant	Ephedra (Ma Huang), Guarana, Kola Nut,
Stomach/Intestinal Problems	Ginger, DGL (Licorice),Milk Thistle, Turmeric, Valerian (cramps)
Stomatitis (ulcerative)	Chamomile (external)
Strep throat	Echinacea
Stress	American Ginseng, Chamomile, Korean Ginseng, Schisandra, Siberian Ginseng, Suma
Styptic	Horsetail, Nettles
Swelling (see Edema)	Devil's Claw, Dong Quai, Echinacea, Feverfew, Ginkgo Biloba
Systemic Cleanser	Guarana

T

Tendonitis	Nettles
Testical Atrophy	Saw Palmetto
Thrombosis	Chinese Garlic
Thrush	Goldenseal (douche)
Thyroid	Ginseng
Thyroid deficiency	Saw Palmetto
Tingling	Ginkgo Biloba, Gotu Kola
Tinnitus	Ginkgo Biloba
Tonsillitis	Echinacea
Toxins	Milk Thistle, Siberian Ginseng
Tranquilizing (see sedative)	American Ginseng

U

Ulcers	Chamomile, Echinacea, Goldenseal, Gotu Kola, Horsetail, Licorice, St. John's Wort
Upset Stomach	Devil's Claw
Urethritis	Goldenseal
Urinary Stones	Horsetail
Urinary Tract	St. John's Wort, Uva Ursi

Urinary Tract Infections (UTI)	Echinacea, Saw Palmetto, Uva Ursi, Willow Bark
Urination, painful	Pygeum, Uva Ursi
Urine Retention	Pygeum
Urticaria	Echinacea, Ephedra (Ma Huang)
Uterine Tonic	Chamomile, Dong Quai, Milk Thistle
Uterine disturbances	Goldenseal

V

Vaginitis	Goldenseal (douche)
Vampires	Chinese Garlic
Varicose Veins, Varices	Bilberry, Butcher's Broom, Grape Seed Extract, Milk Thistle
Vascular disorders	Bilberry, Butcher's Broom, Ginkgo Biloba, Hawthorne
Vertigo	Feverfew, Ginger, Ginkgo Biloba
Vision	Bilberry, Schisandra
Visual fatigue	Bilberry, Schisandra
Vitality (poor)	Dong Quai, Korean Ginseng, Siberian Ginseng
Vomiting	Feverfew, Ginger
Vulnerary	Chamomile (external), Chinese Garlic, Echinacea, St. John's Wort

W

Water retention	Devil's Claw, Echinacea
Weakness	American Ginseng
Weight Loss	Turmeric
Whole Body Tonic	Astragalus, Chamomile, Gotu Kola, Korean Ginseng, Saw Palmetto
Worms	Chinese Garlic, Goldenseal, Willow Bark
Wound healing and cleaning	Chinese Garlic, Echinacea, Nettles, St. John's Wort

Y

Yeast Infections	Echinacea, Turmeric

CNS depressant	Climacteric disorders	Cirrhosis	Circulation	Cholesterol regulation	Cholesterol (high)	Cholalogue	Chills	Chapped skin	Cerebral vascular insufficiency	Cellulitis	Cellulite	Cathartic	Catarrhal conditions	Cataracts	Capillary fragility	Candida (douche)	Cancer preventative	Calming agent	Burn healing	Bronchitis	Bronchodilator	Bone-Flesh-Cartilage	Boils	Blood thinner	Blood sugar regulation	Blood sugar (high/low)	Blood purpuras	Blood purification & detoxification	Blood pressure (high)	Blood clotting	Bladder stones	Bile secretions	Birth Process	Benign Prostate Hypertrophy	Behavioral Disorders	Bedwetting	Bed sores	Atherosclerosis	Astringent	
																																	X							Agnus Castus
X																										X														American Ginseng
				X																												X						X		Artichoke
			X																																					Astragalus
			X											X	X												X												X	Bilberry
			X																																				X	Butcher's Broom
						X						X																												Cascara Sagrada
								X										X																						Chamomile
			X		X															X						X			X											Chinese Garlic
																											X	X												Devil's Claw
					X																																	X		Dong Quai
																							X					X												Echinacea
			X				X														X																			Ephedra (MA Huang)
																																								Feverfew
					X																			X																Ginger
			X						X																															Ginkgo Biloba
													X			X				X									X											Goldenseal
			X							X	X											X															X			Gota Kola
									X						X																									Grape Seed Extract
					X																								X											Green Tea Extract
																																								Guarana
			X																										X											Hawthorne
X																																								Hops
																																							X	Horsetail
																																								Kava Kava
																																								Kola Nut
			X		X																								X											Korean Ginseng
		X																		X					X															Licorice
			X			X																								X										Milk Thistle
																										X								X						Nettles
																																								Passion Flower
																																		X						Pygeum
					X																																			Reishi Mushroom
													X							X														X						Saw Palmetto
																																								Schisandra
		X			X												X																							Shiitake Mushroom
																										X														Siberian Ginseng
																			X																X					St. John's Wort
																																								Suma
				X		X											X															X								Turmeric
																															X								X	Uva Ursi
																													X							X				Valerian
																							X																X	Willow Bark

	Astigmatism	Asthma	Arthritis	Arteriosclerosis	Arterial spasms	Arterial disorders	Appetite reducer	Appetite (loss)	Aphrodisiac	Anxiety	Anti-viral	Anti-toxin	Anti-spasmodic	Antiseptic	Anti-phlogisitic	Antioxidant	Anti-inflammatory	Anti-fungal	Anti-convulsant	Anti-coagulant	Anti-cancer	Anti-bacterial	Antibiotic	Anodyne	Angina	Anemia	Anaphrodesiac	Analgesic	Anal Fissures	Amenorrhea	Alzheimer's	Allergies	Allergic Rhinitis	Allergic exanthemas	AIDS	Aging (vascular problems)	Adrenal Cortex stimulation	Addison's Disease	Adematous fibrosclerosis	Adaptogen	Abcesses	Abrasions
Agnus Castus																														X												
American Ginseng								X					X							X										X										X		
Artichoke			X																																							
Astragalus																																										
Bilberry																																										
Butcher's Broom																														X												
Cascara Sagrada																							X	X																		
Chamomile											X		X	X	X		X					X	X	X	X					X		X										X
Chinese Garlic											X	X						X				X	X	X																	X	
Devil's Claw		X									X	X																		X	X											
Dong Quai				X									X																	X		X										
Echinacea				X									X					X				X	X	X								X					X					X
Ephedra (MA Huang)						X							X					X				X	X	X								X	X									
Feverfew		X				X																																				
Ginger		X	X					X																																		
Ginkgo Biloba																				X																						
Goldenseal		X																					X	X																		
Gota Kola															X																											
Grape Seed Extract						X																														X						
Green Tea Extract																X	X																									
Guarana																	X	X			X																					
Hawthorne						X		X																	X											X						
Hops				X	X					X																																
Horsetail								X		X																	X															
Kava Kava																											X															
Kola Nut				X																																						
Korean Ginseng								X									X																				X	X		X		
Licorice																							X	X													X	X				
Milk Thistle														X																												
Nettles																										X							X	X								
Passion Flower			X																											X												
Pygeum		X										X	X							X																						
Reishi Mushroom																																								X		
Saw Palmetto																																				X						
Schisandra			X					X											X																							
Shiitake Mushroom	X											X	X				X			X			X	X																		X
Siberian Ginseng													X					X	X			X																				
St. John's Wort													X								X																X					
Suma											X	X																														
Turmeric																	X	X																								
Uva Ursi			X														X																									
Valerian										X			X																													
Willow Bark			X																									X														

93

Herb	Endometriosis	Emmenagogue	Edema	Eczema	Ear infections	Dysuria	Dyspepsia	Dysentery	Dysmenorrhea	Dry skin	Dizziness	Diverticulitis	Diuretic	Digestion	Diarrhea	Diaphoretic	Diabetic vascular complications	Diabetic retinopathy	Diabetic induced cataracts	Diabetes	Detoxify	Dermatitis	Depression	Dementia	Debility	Dandruff	Cystitis	Cuts	Crohn's disease	Cough	Cortisol release	Convalescence	Constipation	Connective tissue disorders	Confinement	Concentration	Colds	CNS vascular disturbances	CNS stimulant
Agnus Castus	X								X																														
American Ginseng														X						X					X							X							
Artichoke														X																									
Astragalus																																							
Bilberry																	X	X	X																			X	
Butcher's Broom																		X	X																				
Cascara Sagrada			X							X		X				X						X				X													
Chamomile								X						X														X									X		
Chinese Garlic							X							X																							X		
Devil's Claw			X				X							X																									
Dong Quai			X	X					X																X														
Echinacea			X		X																X									X		X					X		
Ephedra (MA Huang)													X																										
Feverfew		X												X									X																
Ginger							X							X																									
Ginkgo Biloba			X								X									X				X															
Goldenseal			X	X			X							X	X																								
Gota Kola			X																	X														X					
Grape Seed Extract			X																	X																			
Green Tea Extract																																							
Guarana														X	X																								X
Hawthorne														X	X																								
Hops													X	X														X											
Horsetail													X	X											X	X													
Kava Kava																																							
Kola Nut																																							X
Korean Ginseng																																							X
Licorice														X											X							X							
Milk Thistle																																							
Nettles				X									X												X							X							
Passion Flower																																		X					
Pygeum						X																																	
Reishi Mushroom														X																				X					
Saw Palmetto														X																							X		
Schisandra									X					X																							X		
Shiitake Mushroom																				X																			
Siberian Ginseng																								X	X							X					X		
St. John's Wort									X				X												X														
Suma																																							
Turmeric														X																									
Uva Ursi															X												X												
Valerian							X																		X														
Willow Bark								X						X																				X					

Herb	Hyperglycemia	Hyperactivity	High blood pressure	High altitude sickness	Hepatoprotective	Hepatitis	Hemorrhoids	Hemorrhages	Heartburn	Heartbeats (irregular)	Heart tonic	Headaches	Hair (lifeless,loss)	Gums (inflamed)	Gums (bleeding)	Gout	Gonorrhea	Gingivitis	Gastrointestinal problems	Gastritis	Gangrene	Gall Bladder problems	Flu	Flatulence	Fever (acute)	Fertility (male)	Female tonic	Fear (excessive)	Fatigue	Eyes	Eye infections	Expectorant	Exhaustion	Erysepilas	Erectile dysfunction	Episiotomy tears	Epilepsy	Environmental pollution	Enuresis	Endurance
Agnus Castus																																								
American Ginseng																			X						X		X		X											
Artichoke																																								
Astragalus																																								
Bilberry							X	X			X				X																X									
Butcher's Broom							X	X			X																													
Cascara Sagrada																																								
Chamomile									X									X		X				X																
Chinese Garlic																				X			X									X								
Devil's Claw																X						X																		
Dong Quai			X																																					
Echinacea														X	X						X		X										X							
Ephedra (MA Huang)																																							X	
Feverfew												X													X															
Ginger																								X																
Ginkgo Biloba				X							X	X									X														X					
Goldenseal								X	X								X		X	X		X			X															
Gota Kola								X			X																X		X				X		X					
Grape Seed Extract																																								
Green Tea Extract			X																																					
Guarana												X																					X							
Hawthorne										X	X																													
Hops																																								
Horsetail													X																											
Kava Kava												X																												
Kola Nut																													X											
Korean Ginseng																										X							X		X					
Licorice																											X													
Milk Thistle					X	X																X																		
Nettles													X				X																X							
Passion Flower			X					X																																
Pygeum								X																																
Reishi Mushroom			X		X																																			
Saw Palmetto																																X							X	
Schisandra																															X									X
Shiitake Mushroom																																								
Siberian Ginseng																													X											
St. John's Wort	X																											X												
Suma																			X	X																				
Turmeric																						X																		
Uva Ursi									X	X																														
Valerian		X								X																							X				X			
Willow Bark												X	X				X								X															

95

Morning sickness	Migraines	Mental alertness	Mental problems	Menstrual cramps	Menopause	Memory	Mania	Lung complaints	Lumbago	Liver (fatty degeneration)	Liver disorders	Libido (low)	Learning	Laxative	Lactation	Kidney Stones	Kidney Hematuria	Kidney & Liver disorders	Jaundice	Ischemia	Irritable Bowel syndrome	Intermittent Claudication	Insomnia	Influenza	Inflammatory Bowel disorders	Inflammation	Infertility	Infections	Indigestion	Incontinence	Impotence	Imetigo	Immunostimulatory	Immune system	Hysteria	Hypoxia	Hypotension	Hypertension	Hypoglycemia	
			X		X																		X		X	X							X						X	Agnus Castus
											X							X															X					X		American Ginseng
																																								Artichoke
																												X						X				X		Astragalus
																	X																					X		Bilberry
			X																																					Butcher's Broom
											X			X																										Cascara Sagrada
																							X		X	X														Chamomile
				X							X																	X												Chinese Garlic
											X	X						X									X						X	X						Devil's Claw
			X	X	X						X											X				X							X	X						Dong Quai
																						X			X			X					X	X						Echinacea
																																				X				Ephedra (MA Huang)
X	X		X								X												X			X														Feverfew
	X	X				X																																		Ginger
	X	X									X									X					X	X				X							X			Ginkgo Biloba
		X									X															X	X				X									Goldenseal
		X				X							X													X														Gota Kola
																																								Grape Seed Extract
																																								Green Tea Extract
																																								Guarana
																							X		X	X												X		Hawthorne
															X						X	X	X		X	X														Hops
							X																								X	X								Horsetail
																																								Kava Kava
																																								Kola Nut
		X																					X					X					X	X						Korean Ginseng
											X			X											X	X				X									X	Licorice
				X						X	X			X			X		X																					Milk Thistle
			X						X						X										X															Nettles
		X	X		X																		X			X														Passion Flower
																														X										Pygeum
						X																	X			X							X							Reishi Mushroom
			X	X											X			X								X				X										Saw Palmetto
	X				X						X					X	X		X		X					X								X			X			Schisandra
	X																						X		X	X							X	X						Shiitake Mushroom
				X		X																	X				X	X					X	X				X		Siberian Ginseng
											X														X	X											X			St. John's Wort
																																								Suma
			X							X																			X											Turmeric
			X													X	X																							Uva Ursi
			X																			X	X																	Valerian
			X																							X														Willow Bark

Pregnancy lesions	Pregnancy cramps	Post thrombotic syndrome	Polyuria	Polynephritis	Pollution	Pneumonia	PMS	Pigmentary retinitis	Physical performance	Phlebitis	Pharyngitis	Peripheral Vascular Disease	Peripheral Arterial Insufficiency	Perineal lesions during delivery	Parturition	Parasites	Paradentosis	Pancreatic tonic	Palpitations	Pain relief	Ovarian function	Obesity	Nycturia	Numbness	Nocturnal cramps	Nightmares	Night vision	Neurasthenia	Neuralgia	Nervous tension	Nervous breakdown	Nephritis	Near-sightedness	Nausea	Nasal congestion	Nails	Myopia	Myasthenia gravis	Myalgias	Muscles (sore)	Motion sickness	Herb
							X																																			Agnus Castus
																														X												American Ginseng
																																										Artichoke
																																								X		Astragalus
								X			X																X										X					Bilberry
X	X																																									Butcher's Broom
																																										Cascara Sagrada
											X						X	X												X												Chamomile
						X										X																										Chinese Garlic
																																										Devil's Claw
							X					X									X																					Dong Quai
																					X														X							Echinacea
																					X																					Ephedra (MA Huang)
																																		X								Feverfew
																																		X							X	Ginger
												X	X											X						X												Ginkgo Biloba
																	X																									Goldenseal
X										X				X											X																	Gota Kola
													X																													Grape Seed Extract
																																										Green Tea Extract
																					X										X											Guarana
																															X											Hawthorne
																															X											Hops
																																				X						Horsetail
																																										Kava Kava
																																										Kola Nut
									X																					X												Korean Ginseng
																																										Licorice
																																										Milk Thistle
																																										Nettles
															X															X												Passion Flower
			X																				X																			Pygeum
																																										Reishi Mushroom
																				X		X																				Saw Palmetto
																			X									X						X								Schisandra
																																										Shiitake Mushroom
						X			X																					X	X											Siberian Ginseng
																													X	X	X									X		St. John's Wort
																																										Suma
																							X												X							Turmeric
			X																														X									Uva Ursi
																			X												X											Valerian
																	X				X																			X	X	Willow Bark

Reference grid — herbs (rows) and ailments/uses (columns). An "X" marks a listed use.

Herb	Stomatitis	Stomach-Intestinal problems	Strep throat	Stimulant	Sterility	Spondylosis-induced lower back pain	Spleen tonic	Spastic colon	Sore throats	Sores	Snakebites	Skin injuries	Skin infections	Skin disorders	Skin (chapped)	Sinusitis	Sinus congestion	Shampoo	Sedative	Sciatica	Ringworm	Rhinitis	Rheumatism	Retinal disturbances	Restorative	Restlessness	Respiratory ailments	Respiratory inflammations	Relaxation	Rectal inflammations	Raynaud's syndrome	Rashes	Radioprotective	Purgative	Pulmonary Tuberculosis	Psychosis	Psoriasis	Pruritis ani (anal itching)	Proteinuria	Prostate problems	Prostate cancer	Proctology	Proctitis
Agnus Castus																			X										X								X						
American Ginseng																																											
Artichoke																																							X				
Astragalus																																											
Bilberry														X										X																			
Butcher's Broom													X	X										X													X					X	X
Cascara Sagrada																																		X									
Chamomile	X									X					X				X							X			X														
Chinese Garlic																																											
Devil's Claw						X													X				X																				
Dong Quai																			X																								
Echinacea			X						X	X	X			X					X									X															
Ephedra (MA Huang)				X																								X															
Feverfew																			X							X																	
Ginger		X																																									
Ginkgo Biloba																															X												
Goldenseal													X	X					X		X	X								X													
Gota Kola										X		X	X	X																													
Grape Seed Extract																								X																			
Green Tea Extract																												X															
Guarana				X																																							
Hawthorne																															X												
Hops																			X							X																	
Horsetail														X				X																	X					X			
Kava Kava																			X										X														
Kola Nut				X																																							
Korean Ginseng																									X								X							X			
Licorice	X																														X												
Milk Thistle							X																														X						
Nettles																X	X			X		X																		X			
Passion Flower																			X																								
Pygeum																																								X	X		
Reishi Mushroom																																	X										
Saw Palmetto																			X																					X			
Schisandra																																											
Shiitake Mushroom																																											
Siberian Ginseng					X																																						
St. John's Wort																			X	X															X								
Suma																									X																		
Turmeric	X																																							X			
Uva Ursi																																											
Valerian	X							X																		X																	
Willow Bark																							X																				

Herb	Yeast infections	Wound healing / cleaning	Worms	Whole body tonic	Weight loss	Weakness	Water retention	Vulnerary	Vomiting	Vitality (poor)	Visual fatigue	Vision	Vertigo	Vascular disorders	Varicose veins	Vampires	Vaginitis (douches)	Uterine tonic	Uterine disturbances	Urticaria	Urinary tract infections	Urinary stones	Urine retention	Urination (painful)	Urethritis	Upset Stomach	Ulcers	Tranquilizing	Toxins	Tonsilitis	Tinnitus	Tingling	Thyroid deficiency	Thyroid	Thrush (douche)	Thrombosis	Testical atrophy	Tendonitis	Systemic cleanser	Swelling	Styptic	Stress
Agnus Castus																																										
American Ginseng						X																						X						X								X
Artichoke																																										
Astragalus				X																																						
Bilberry											X	X		X	X																											
Butcher's Broom														X	X																											
Cascara Sagrada																																										
Chamomile									X									X									X															X
Chinese Garlic			X						X								X																			X						
Devil's Claw								X																		X														X		
Dong Quai										X								X																						X		
Echinacea	X	X					X	X												X	X						X			X										X		
Ephedra																				X																						
Feverfew														X																										X		
Ginger													X	X																												
Ginkgo Biloba													X	X																	X	X								X		
Goldenseal			X														X		X						X		X								X							
Gota Kola																											X			X												
Grape Seed Extract														X	X																											
Green Tea Extract																																										
Guarana																																							X			
Hawthorne														X																												
Hops																																										
Horsetail																						X					X														X	
Kava Kava																																										
Kola Nut																																										
Korean Ginseng				X						X																								X								X
Licorice																											X															
Milk Thistle																													X													
Nettles																																						X		X		
Passion Flower			X																																							
Pygeum																							X	X																		
Reishi Mushroom																																										
Saw Palmetto																					X												X		X							
Schisandra												X	X																													X
Shiitake Mushroom																																										
Siberian Ginseng											X																		X					X								X
St. John's Wort			X					X																			X															
Suma																																										X
Turmeric	X					X																																				
Uva Ursi																					X		X																			
Valerian																																										
Willow Bark			X																		X																					

99

For additional information on Herbal Products, contact the following organizations:

American Botanical Council
P.O. Box 201660,
Austin, TX 78720
(512) 331-8868
FAX (512) 331-1924

Herb Research Foundation
1007 Pearl Street, Suite 200
Boulder, CO 80302
(303) 449-2265
FAX (303) 449-7849